Community Health Nursing Test Success

Frances H. Cornelius, PhD, MSN, RN-BC, CNE, is associate clinical professor, chair of the MSN Advanced Practice Role Department and coordinator of informatics projects at Drexel University, College of Nursing and Health Professions. Frances has taught nursing since 1991, at several schools of nursing. She taught community health at Madonna University (Livonia, MI), Oakland (MI) University, University of Pittsburgh (PA), and Holy Family College (Philadelphia, PA). Frances taught adult health and gerontology at Widener University School of Nursing until 1997, when she began teaching at Drexel. In 2003, she was a fellow at the Biomedical Library of Medicine. She is a certified nurse informaticist and has been the recipient of several grants. She has collaborated on the development of mobile applications as coordinator of informatics projects, including the Patient Assessment and Care Plan Development (PACPD) tool, which is a PDA tool with a web-based companion, and Gerontology Reasoning Informatics Programs (the GRIP project). She is the coeditor (with Mary Gallagher Gordon) of *PDA Connections*, an innovative textbook designed to teach health care professionals how to use mobile devices for point-of-care access of information. She has written six book chapters and has published 19 journal articles on her work. She has been invited to deliver 26 presentations and has delivered more than 50 peer-reviewed presentations mostly in the United States, but also in Spain, Canada, and Korea. She is a member of the American Informatics Association, the American Nursing Informatics Association, the American Nurses Association, and the Pennsylvania State Nurses Association.

Ruth A. Wittmann-Price, PhD, RN, CNS, CNE, is chairperson and professor at Francis Marion University Department of Nursing in South Carolina. Ruth has been an obstetrical/women's health nurse for 35 years. She received her AAS and BSN degrees from Felician College in Lodi, NJ (1978, 1981), and her MS as a perinatal CNS from Columbia University, NY (1983). Ruth completed her PhD at Widener University, Chester, PA (2006), and was awarded the Dean's Award for Excellence. She developed a mid-range nursing theory "Emancipated Decision-Making in Women's Health Care." Besides continuing her research about decisional science, she studies developmental outcomes of preterm infants. She has also been the director of nursing research for Hahnemann University Hospital (2007–2010) and oversees all evidence-based practice projects for nursing. Hahnemann University Hospital was awarded initial Magnet status (American Nurses Credentialing Center) in December 2009. Ruth has taught all levels of nursing students over the past 15 years (AAS, BSN, MSN, and DNP) and completed an international service learning trip (2007) to rural Mexico with undergraduate nursing and physician assistant students. She was the coordinator for the nurse educator track in the DrNP program at Drexel University in Philadelphia (2007–2010) and sits on four dissertation committees. Ruth is coeditor and chapter contributor of six books, *Nursing Education: Foundations for Practice Excellence* (2007) (AJN Book of the Year Award winner 2007); *The Certified Nurse Examination (CNE) Review Manual* (2012); *NCLEX-RN® EXCEL Test Success Through Unfolding Case Study Review; Maternal-Child Nursing Test Success: An Unfolding Case Study Review* (2012); *Fundamentals of Nursing Test Success: An Unfolding Case Study Review* (2013); and *Nursing Concept Care Maps for Safe Patient Care* (2013). She has published the chapter "The Newborn at Risk" in *Maternal-Child Nursing Care: Optimizing Outcomes for Mothers, Children, and Families*, a section in *Giving Through Teaching: How Nurse Educators Are Changing the World*, and over 20 journal articles.

Community Health Nursing Test Success: An Unfolding Case Study Review

Frances H. Cornelius, PhD, MSN, RN-BC, CNE
Ruth A. Wittmann-Price, PhD, RN, CNS, CNE

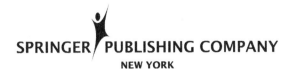

SPRINGER PUBLISHING COMPANY
NEW YORK

Springer Publishing Company, LLC
11 West 42nd Street
New York, NY 10036
www.springerpub.com

Acquisitions Editor: Margaret Zuccarini
Composition: S4Carlisle Publishing Services

ISBN: 978-0-8261-1013-8
E-book ISBN: 978-0-8261-1003-9
eResources ISBN: 978-0-8261-7133-7

A list of eResources is available from www.springerpub.com/cornelius-ancillaries

13 14 15 / 5 4 3 2 1

The author and the publisher of this Work have made every effort to use sources believed to be reliable to provide information that is accurate and compatible with the standards generally accepted at the time of publication. Because medical science is continually advancing, our knowledge base continues to expand. Therefore, as new information becomes available, changes in procedures become necessary. We recommend that the reader always consult current research and specific institutional policies before performing any clinical procedure. The author and publisher shall not be liable for any special, consequential, or exemplary damages resulting, in whole or in part, from the readers' use of, or reliance on, the information contained in this book. The publisher has no responsibility for the persistence or accuracy of URLs for external or third-party Internet websites referred to in this publication and does not guarantee that any content on such websites is, or will remain, accurate or appropriate.

Library of Congress Cataloging-in-Publication Data

Cornelius, Frances H.
  Community health nursing test success : an unfolding case study review / Frances H. Cornelius, Ruth A. Wittmann-Price.
    p. ; cm.
  Includes bibliographical references and index.
  ISBN 978-0-8261-1013-8—ISBN 0-8261-1013-4—ISBN 978-0-8261-1003-9 (e-book)
  I. Wittmann-Price, Ruth A. II. Title.
    [DNLM: 1. Community Health Nursing—Case Reports. 2. Community Health Nursing—Problems and Exercises. 3. Nursing Care—Case Reports. 4. Nursing Care—Problems and Exercises. 5. Test Taking Skills—methods. WY 18.2]
  362.14—dc23   2012049529

Printed in the United States of America by Bradford & Bigelow.

*To our families, friends, and colleagues—
sources of strength and inspiration*

Contents

Preface

Community health nursing is becoming more and more important due to increasing outpatient and home health care. This book was designed for learners and nurse educators as a unique way to present community health nursing content. It uses a successful, innovative format and is one of the unfolding case study books in this review series. Unfolding case studies with embedded NCLEX-style questions increase learner comprehension and simulate real-life nursing situations. This book can be used effectively in a number of ways. Learners can use this book as a tool to better comprehend community nursing content or review for the NCLEX exam. Nurse educators love to use this book to mentor and coach learners or assign as an alternative learning strategy when a learner needs to make up clinical time or needs extra remediation in a particular area.

This book engages users in *active learning* using *unfolding case studies*. Unfolding case studies differ from traditional case studies because they evolve over time. Billings, Kowalski, and Reese (2011) describe unfolding case studies as a method to help "clinical reasoning and independent thinking skills" (p. 344). Unfolding case studies assist the learner to problem-solve and understand content on a deeper level (Day, 2011; Page, Kowlowitz, & Alden, 2010).

Unlike other NCLEX review books, this book builds content and evaluation right into the case scenarios, facilitating active learning as students are working through the compelling and increasingly more complex unfolding case studies. Over 200 NCLEX-style questions are embedded in the cases to evaluate learning as the case unfolds. Questions include true or false, multiple choice, matching, select all that apply, chart exhibit format, and fill in the blank. The personalization of patient care content stimulates clinical reasoning and decision making unlike answering question after question in isolation.

In addition to the plentiful NCLEX-style questions, appropriate web links and resources are incorporated into the unfolding cases as a means to further replicate realistic clinical situations in which the point-of-care/point-of-need access to information is utilized for clinical decision support. Mobile resources such as PubMed and Agency for Healthcare Research and Quality guidelines as well as others are utilized for this purpose. For example, in the case study involving a home visit, the eResources would likely include links to:

1. A brief video clip from YouTube regarding home safety
2. The Electronic Preventive Services Selector for health assessments
3. Mobile device resources for patient drug or laboratory data pertinent to the case

Also interwoven in the unfolding cases are the current Quality and Safety Education for Nurses (QSEN) competencies: patient-centered care, teamwork and collaboration, evidence-based practice, quality improvement, safety, and informatics. Using QSEN as a framework, the cases take on real-life situations that occur in current clinical practice. This unique book encourages learners to "think like" a community health nurse who is problem solving in the field.

We are confident that you will find this book an amazing learning tool and will enjoy the self-paced comprehensive features that make it so different from other review books. Understanding community health principles and content will become increasingly important for today's health care system, and this book will provide you with the advantage you need to master that content in an exciting new way!

Frances H. Cornelius, PhD, MSN, RN-BC, CNE
Ruth A. Wittmann-Price, PhD, RN, CNS, CNE

References

Billings, D. M., Kowalski, K., & Reese, C. E. (2011). Unfolding case studies. *Journal of Continuing Nursing Education, 42*(8), 344–345.

Day, L. (2011). Unfolding case studies in a subject-centered classroom. *Journal of Nursing Education, 50*(8), 447–452.

Page, J. B., Kowlowitz, V., & Alden, K. R. (2010). Development of a scripted unfolding case study focusing on delirium in older adults. *Journal of Continuing Nursing Education, 41*(5), 225–230.

Acknowledgments

We would like to acknowledge the support and patience of our publishers, particularly Margaret Zuccarini.

Nursing Test Success

With Ruth A. Wittmann-Price as Series Editor

Maternal-Child Nursing Test Success: An Unfolding Case Study Review
Ruth A. Wittmann-Price, PhD, RN, CNS, CNE, and
Frances H. Cornelius, PhD, MSN, RN-BC, CNE

Fundamentals of Nursing Test Success: An Unfolding Case Study Review
Ruth A. Wittmann-Price, PhD, RN, CNS, CNE, and
Frances H. Cornelius, PhD, MSN, RN-BC, CNE

Community Health Nursing Test Success: An Unfolding Case Study Review
Frances H. Cornelius, PhD, MSN, RN-BC, CNE, and
Ruth A. Wittmann-Price, PhD, RN, CNS, CNE

Medical-Surgical Nursing Test Success: An Unfolding Case Study Review
Karen K. Gittings, DNP, RN, CNE, Alumnus CCRN, Rhonda M. Brogdon, DNP, MSN, MBA, RN, and Frances H. Cornelius, PhD, MSN, RN-BC, CNE

Leadership and Management in Nursing Test Success: An Unfolding Case Study Review
Ruth A. Wittmann-Price, PhD, RN, CNS, CNE, and
Frances H. Cornelius, PhD, MSN, RN-BC, CNE

1

Introduction to Community/Public Health Nursing

Sally, Abigail, and Rick are senior nursing students who have just started taking their Community/Public Health Nursing course. To introduce the class to the broad concepts of community/public health nursing, their instructor has arranged to have a panel of nurses who are working in a variety of settings discuss the wide variety of roles nursing can serve in the community. To prepare the students for the panel presentation, she reviews with them the concepts related to community and public health nursing. She begins by asking the class, "What is a community? What are the characteristics of a community?"

Exercise 1-1: *Fill-in*
Enter your definition of community:

_____

_____

List the characteristics of a community:

_____

_____

In addition, the instructor tells the class that many nurses work in the community, but the focus of their work differs—some are population-focused while others are community-oriented.

Exercise 1-2: *Multiple-choice question*
Which of the following definitions best describes population-focused nursing?
- A. Focuses care on individuals, families, and groups to help manage both acute and chronic health issues across the life span in community or home settings
- B. Focuses on the health of an entire family, identification of actual or potential health concerns, and implementation and evaluation of needed interventions to maintain health
- C. Focus is on improving the health and health outcomes of one or more populations
- D. Approach in which individuals and their families/significant others are considered integral components of the decision-making and care delivery processes

Answers to this chapter begin on page 13.

The instructor brings in the guest speakers and introduces them to the class. The four-member panel consists of:

- David Hadden, BSN, RN, who works at the city health department
- Warren West, MSN, NCSN, RN, who works as a school nurse
- Donna Atkins, BSN, RN, who works in home care
- Allison Porter, MSN, RN, who works in occupational health

After introducing the panel, each member describes his or her current practice setting, role, and responsibilities. Sally raises her hand and asks the panel, "What is the difference between community health nursing (CHN) and public health nursing (PHN)? It seems to me that the terms are often used interchangeably. Can you please explain this to us?"

David responds that historically both CHNs and PHNs were similar in that they provided care outside of hospitals, and the trend is that more and more care is being delivered outside of the hospitals or long-term care facilities. But, he goes on to explain, not all care given in the community is really public health. The best way to understand the difference between public health and community-based nursing is to look at how the nurse is practicing—specifically the setting and approach—and, of course, the skills required.

Donna further explains by telling the students that "the term 'community health nurse' is … an umbrella term used for all nurses who work in a community, including those who have formal preparation in public health nursing. In essence, public health nursing requires specific educational preparation, and community health nursing denotes a setting for the practice of nursing" (U.S. Department of Health and Human Services [USDHHS], 1985, p. 4).

The students remained somewhat confused regarding the differences between community nursing and public health nursing. So the panel provides a series of examples of CHN and PHN practice activities.

Exercise 1-3: *Fill-in*

Decide which of the following activities below are examples of public health nursing (PHN) activities or community health nursing (CHN) activities. [Enter a **P** for PHN and a **C** for CHN]

_____ Nurse evaluates health trends and risk factors of a population and helps to identify priorities for directed interventions.

_____ Nurse works with communities to develop public policy and focused health promotion and disease prevention activities.

_____ Nurse conducts interviews and takes family histories to collect and analyze the information about the family system (e.g., family development, structure and function, communication patterns) to identify family support needs and link with available community services.

Answers to this chapter begin on page 13.

_____ Nurse participates in assessment and evaluation of health care services to promote awareness of and provide assistance in accessing those services.

_____ Nurse uses the nursing process to maximize the strength of the individual while incorporating the community in efforts to facilitate wellness.

_____ Nurse provides essential input to interdisciplinary programs that monitor, anticipate, and respond to public health problems in population groups.

_____ Nurse provides health education, care management, and primary care to individuals and families who are members of vulnerable population and high-risk groups.

_____ Nurse provides direct care for individuals, families, and groups outside of an institution, such as in home care services to a high-risk infant.

Exercise 1-4: *Fill-in*

The class is starting to understand these concepts. Abigail raises her hand and says, "Okay, I think I have it now."

Community-based nursing is:

_____

Community-oriented nursing is:

_____

To help the class understand the terms better, the panel provides additional examples of community-based nursing and community-oriented nursing.

Exercise 1-5: *Matching*

Match the following characteristics with either community-based (CB) or community-oriented (CO) nursing.

_____ Population focused

_____ Public health nursing

_____ Involves practice within a certain setting

_____ Home health care nursing

_____ Requires a greater cognizance of the connections of various factors with health

_____ Involves ensuring ease of access to competent nursing services

Answers to this chapter begin on page 13.

_____ Involves the delivery of nursing care to individuals and families who are "ill"

_____ Involves community diagnosis

_____ Involves the delivery of acute and chronic care to individuals and families in a specific setting

_____ Occupational health nursing

_____ Hospice nursing

To further clarify the differences between community-oriented nursing and community-based nursing, the instructor asks the class some more questions.

Exercise 1-6: *Multiple-choice question*
"Illness care" is characteristic of:

        A. Community-oriented nursing

        B. Public health nursing

        C. Community-based nursing

        D. All of the above

Warren West, the school nurse, provides additional insights by telling the class, "You need to look at what the focus of care is. For example, a school nurse is responsible for (a) doing routine health assessments and (b) providing medications for children with asthma, diabetes, or seizures."

Exercise 1-7: *Multiple-choice question*
These activities are characteristic of:

        A. Community-based nursing

        B. Community-oriented nursing

        C. Population-based nursing

        D. Both A and B

The instructor also wanted to use the panel discussion to heighten student understanding of the Scope and Standards of Practice for Pubic Health Nursing (PHN) as well as the essential competencies required of the nurse. She asks the students to think about the Scope and Standards of Practice for Nursing and compare these with those of PHN.

Exercise 1-8: *Fill-in*
Look at the table on the next page, which lists the ANA Nursing and PHN Scope and Standards of Practice. Using the ANA publications as a reference, identify the similarities and differences between the two. Discuss the differences. Identify the similarities and differences between the two. Discuss the differences.

Sally raises her hand and asks, "We have learned throughout our nursing program that the nurse's role is to be an advocate for his/her patient. Why isn't 'Advocacy' listed as a standard for ANA's Nursing Scope and Standards of Practice?" The instructor replies,

Answers to this chapter begin on page 13.

Table 1-1: Comparison of ANA Nursing and PHN Scope and Standards of Practice

Nursing	Public Health Nursing	Notes
Standard 1—Assessment	Standard 1—Assessment	
Standard 2—Diagnosis	Standard 2—Population Diagnosis and Priorities	
Standard 3—Outcomes Identification		
Standard 4—Planning	Standard 3—Outcomes Identification	
Standard 5—Implementation	Standard 4—Planning	
Standard 5a—Coordination of Care	Standard 5—Implementation	
Standard 5b—Health Teaching and Health Promotion	Standard 5a—Coordination of Care	
Standard 5c—Consultation	Standard 5b—Health Education and Health Promotion	
Standard 5d—Prescriptive Authority and Treatment	Standard 5c—Consultation	
Standard 6—Evaluation	Standard 5d—Regulatory Activities	
Standard 7—Quality of Practice	Standard 6—Evaluation	
Standard 8—Education	Standard 7—Quality of Practice	
Standard 9—Professional Practice Evaluation	Standard 8—Education	
Standard 10—Collegiality	Standard 9—Professional Practice Evaluation	
Standard 11—Collaboration	Standard 10—Collegiality and Professional Relationships	
Standard 12—Ethics	Standard 11—Collaboration	
Standard 13—Research	Standard 12—Ethics	
Standard 14—Resource Utilization	Standard 13—Research	
Standard 15—Leadership	Standard 14—Resource Utilization	
	Standard 15—Leadership	
	Standard 16—Advocacy	

Source: ANA (2004, 2007).

"Good question, Sally! You are right. The nurse's role is that of a patient advocate. In the ANA's publication, the responsibility of advocacy is addressed in Standard 12— Ethics where it states that the nurse "serves as a patient advocate assisting patients in

Answers to this chapter begin on page 13.

developing skills for self-advocacy" (ANA, 2004, p. 39). She goes on to ask the class to list other responsibilities of the community/public health nurse.

Exercise 1-9: *Fill-in*
List the responsibilities of the community/public health nurse.

_____

_____

_____

_____

The class moves on to discuss the various ways that nurses can meet these responsibilities in various settings and how these are coordinated with the core functions of public health.

Exercise 1-10: *Fill-in*
What are the core functions of public health?

_____

_____

_____

_____

The instructor goes on to tell the class that there are 10 Essential Public Health Services and these align with the core public health functions.

Exercise 1-11: *Fill-in*
Align the core public health function with the relevant essential public health service (A for Assessment or PD for Policy Development):

Table 1-2

Core Public Health Function	Essential Public Health Services
	1. Monitor health status to identify and solve community health problems
	2. Diagnose and investigate health problems and health hazards in the community
	3. Inform, educate, and empower people about health issues

Answers to this chapter begin on page 13.

Table 1-2 *Continued*

Core Public Health Function	Essential Public Health Services
	4. Mobilize community partnerships and action to identify and solve health problems
	5. Develop policies and plans that support individual and community health efforts
	6. Enforce laws and regulations that protect health and ensure safety
	7. Link people to needed personal health services and ensure the provision of health care when otherwise unavailable
	8 Ensure competent public and personal health care workforce
	9. Evaluate effectiveness, accessibility, and quality of personal and population-based health services
	10. Research for new insights and innovative solutions to health problems

 eResource 1-1: To learn more about specific activities within the essential services, Rick opens the browser on his smartphone and checks out the Indiana Department of Public Health detailed overview: http://goo.gl/Yp4Fc

The instructor points out to the class that in all of these activities, there are ethical issues that must be considered. The instructor asks the students to consider the similarities between the ethical principles of nursing and those of public health. "For example," she says, "both respect autonomy, doing good, avoiding harm, and treating people fairly and with respect."

Exercise 1-12: *Select all that apply*
The principle of autonomy includes which of the following?

    ❏ Protection of privacy

    ❏ Paternalistic approach

    ❏ Respect for the person

    ❏ Informed consent

    ❏ Fulfillment of client goals

    ❏ Egalitarianism

The class reviews some of the other concepts associated with nursing ethics.

Answers to this chapter begin on page 13.

Exercise 1-13: *Matching*

Match the term in column A with the definition in column B.

Column A	Column B
A. Autonomy	_____ Concept that implies that some people are worthy to have a roof over their heads and others are not
B. Nonmaleficence	_____ The condition of being independent and free to make your own decisions
C. Beneficence	_____ To do no harm, an obligation to not intentionally or knowingly inflict harm
D. Distributive justice	_____ Action taken for the benefit of others, to help prevent or remove harm or to improve the situation of others

(e) eResource 1-2: To learn more about these terms, go to the University of California, San Francisco (UCSF) website: http://goo.gl/kCDgQ

The instructor wants to move the discussion to efforts to improve the health of populations. She asks the class to think about factors that influence health.

The class engages in a discussion about health and how health of the population affects the country. The instructor asks the class to consider factors that affect health, "Let's make a list of the things you think are determinants of health."

Exercise 1-14: *Fill-in*

List factors that are determinants of health.

1. _____

2. _____

3. _____

4. _____

5. _____

6. _____

7. _____

Answers to this chapter begin on page 13.

The instructor tells the class that health indicators for various populations in the United States are tracked on an ongoing basis and made available to anyone who is interested in this information. She tells the students that simply knowing the determinants of health is not enough. There must be a mechanism to collect data and disseminate the data to improve insights regarding a community's health status and determinants and that can facilitate the identification and prioritization of interventions.

 eResource 1-3: Health Indicators Warehouse (HIW) http://healthindicators.gov

To help the class understand the factors that influence health, she shows them the Ecological Model of Health.

Figure 1-1: Models of Health

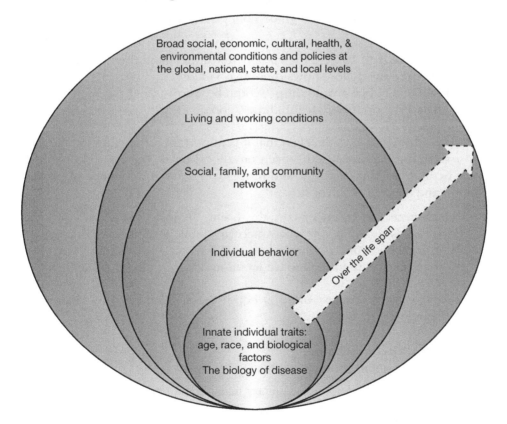

Exercise 1-15: *Multiple-choice question*
One factor is primarily responsible for the differences in health care needs and health care outcomes among various countries. That factor is

    A. Economic development of the country

    B. Political system of the country

Answers to this chapter begin on page 13.

C. Social-cultural system of the country

D. Religious faith of the country's main population

 eResource 1-4: To demonstrate how the economic growth of a country is linked with the health of the nation's population, the instructor shows the class:

- A brief video lecture by Hans Rosling entitled *200 Countries, 200 Years:* http://youtu.be/jbkSRLYSojo
- GapMinder: An interactive tool that permits visualization of the comparison of economic growth and health of select countries: http://goo.gl/p2R3p

The class engages in a lively discussion regarding the factors that influence the health of a nation and how the visual representation of the data collected over time can build understanding and guide policy. The instructor shows them another resource.

 eResource 1-5: To help the class better understand the role of public health, the instructor shows them two videos:
■ What is Public Health: http://youtu.be/ekc5t-ftZoQ
■ The Face of Public Health: http://goo.gl/XEqzR

The instructor points out to the class that it is important for nursing to take a leadership role in the nation's health—even on a local level. There are problems that need to be addressed proactively, and nurses can make a difference in providing education and serving as advocates.

 eResource 1-6: To underscore this point, the instructor shows the class two videos distributed by the American Public Health Association:
■ A Healthier America: http://goo.gl/N3Aj5
■ Healthiest Nation in One Generation: http://youtu.be/ABMSfiozfjg

The class moves on to discuss more in depth the specific activities that a public health nurse may be involved in.

Exercise 1-16: *Select all that apply*

What activities is a public health nurse likely to be involved in?

❏ Collaborate with interdisciplinary teams to monitor and respond to health problems in population groups.

❏ Analyze health trends and risk factors of population groups to define priorities for targeted interventions.

❏ Collaborate with communities to develop targeted health promotion and disease prevention activities.

Answers to this chapter begin on page 13.

❏ Evaluate available health care services.

❏ Provide health education, nursing care, case management, and primary care to vulnerable populations and high-risk groups.

❏ Participate in interdisciplinary programs that monitor, anticipate, and respond to public health problems.

❏ Appraise health trends, patterns, and risk factors of populations.

❏ Collaborate in development of public policy and targeted health promotion and disease prevention activities.

❏ Participate in efforts to disseminate information to promote health and reduce risk.

❏ Serve as an expert consultant on health matters.

❏ Appraise patterns and risk factors that present potential or actual environmental hazards and concerns.

eResource 1-7: To learn more about essential competencies for a public health nurse,

- Sally uses her mobile device to view the Quad Council's Public Health Nurse (PHN) Competencies: [Pathway: www.phnurse.org → select "Resources" → Documents → Current and scroll down to select "Quad Council PHN Competencies 2011"]
- Rick also finds a handout from a presentation at the School of Public Health at the University of Albany, which provides an overview of Public Health Nursing Competencies: http://goo.gl/zyoeR

Sally and Rick share these resources with the class. The instructor remarks that there are a variety of resources available that can help students understand the requisite competencies essential for public health care professionals. She encourages the class to explore these resources. The instructor wants the students to explore competencies more deeply to better understand the value of establishing core competencies.

eResource 1-8: The instructor shows the class a presentation entitled *Core Competencies for Public Health Professionals—Background and Tools* by Ron Bialek, President, Public Health Foundation National: http://goo.gl/C7mPR

After viewing the short presentation, she asks the class the following questions:

Exercise 1-17: *Fill-in*

What is the value of core competencies…

1. To the profession?

_____

_____

Answers to this chapter begin on page 13.

2. To the health care organization?

_____

_____

3. To the public?

_____

_____

Answers to this chapter begin on page 13.

Answers

Exercise 1-1: *Fill-in*

Enter your definition of community:

Oxford Dictionaries definition of community:

1. **A group of people:**
   - **living in the same place or having a particular characteristic in common**
   - **living together and practicing common ownership**
   - **of a district or country considered collectively, especially in the context of social values and responsibilities; society**

2. **The condition of sharing or having certain attitudes and interests in common; a similarity or identity**

   The *American Heritage® Dictionary of the English Language* definition of community:

1. **A group of people:**
   - **living in the same locality and under the same government**
   - **having common interests: the scientific community; the international business community**
   - **viewed as forming a distinct segment of society: the gay community; the community of color**
   - **having similarity or identity: a community of interests**
   - **sharing, participation, and fellowship**

2. **The district or locality in which such a group lives**

3. **Society as a whole; the public**

List the characteristics of a community:

- **Race**
- **Ethnicity**
- **Geographic region**
- **Interests**
- **Gender**
- **Values**
- **Culture**
- **Language**

- **<u>Socioeconomic status</u>**
- **<u>Religious/spiritual preferences</u>**
- **<u>Employment/vocation</u>**
- **<u>Age</u>**
- **<u>Roles</u>**
- **<u>Health issues/concerns (e.g., HIV, diabetes, asthma)</u>**
- **<u>Identity</u>**
- **<u>Political affiliation</u>**

Exercise 1-2: *Multiple-choice question*
Which of the following definition best describes population-focused nursing?
  A. Focuses care on individuals, families, and groups to help manage both acute and chronic health issues across the life span in community or home settings—NO, this focus is on populations.
  B. Focuses on the health of an entire family, identification of actual or potential health concerns, and implementation and evaluation of needed interventions to maintain health—NO, this focus is on populations.
  C. **Focus is upon improving the health and health outcomes of one or more populations—YES, this focus is correct.**
  D. Approach in which individuals and their families/significant others are considered integral components of the decision-making and care delivery processes—NO, this focus is on populations.

Exercise 1-3: *Fill-in*
Decide which of the following activities below are examples of public health nursing (PHN) activities or community health nursing (CHN) activities. [Enter a **P** for PHN and a **C** for CHN]
<u>P</u> Nurse evaluates health trends and risk factors of a population and helps to identify priorities for directed interventions.
<u>P</u> Nurse works with communities to develop public policy and focused health promotion and disease prevention activities.
<u>C</u> Nurse conducts interviews and takes family histories to collect and analyze the information about the family system (e.g., family development, structure and function, communication patterns) to identify family support needs and link with available community services.
<u>P</u> Nurse participates in assessment and evaluation of health care services to promote awareness and provide assistance in accessing those services.
<u>C</u> Nurse uses the nursing process to maximize the strength of the individual while incorporating the community in efforts to facilitate wellness.

P Nurse provides essential input to interdisciplinary programs that monitor, anticipate, and respond to public health problems in population groups.

P Nurse provides health education, care management, and primary care to individuals and families who are members of vulnerable population and high-risk groups.

C Nurse provides direct care for individuals, families, and groups outside of an institution, such as in home care services to a high-risk infant.

Exercise 1-4: *Fill-in*

The class is starting to understand these concepts. Abigail raises her hand and says, "Okay, I think I have it now."

Community-based nursing is when a nurse cares for ill patients *in the* community setting. This is also called "family-centered illness care"; for example, home health nursing.

Community-oriented nursing is when the nurse is focused upon the *health care of individuals, groups, and communities.* This includes *community health* and *public health;* for example, school, parish nursing.

Exercise 1-5: *Matching*

Match the following characteristics with either community-based (CB) or community-oriented (CO) nursing.

CO	Population focused
CO	Public health nursing
CB	Involves practice within a certain setting
CB	Home health care nursing
CO	Requires a greater cognizance of the connections of a variety of factors with health
CO	Involves ensuring ease of access to competent nursing services
CB	Involves the delivery of nursing care to individuals and families who are "ill"
CO	Involves community diagnosis
CB	Involves the delivery of acute and chronic care to individuals and families in a specific setting
CO	Occupational health nursing
CB	Hospice nursing

Exercise 1-6: *Multiple-choice question*

"Illness care" is characteristic of:

A. Community-oriented nursing—NO, it is community-based.

B. Public health nursing—NO, it is community-based.

C. Community-based nursing—YES

D. All of the above—NO, it is community-based only.

Exercise 1-7: *Multiple-choice question*

These activities are characteristic of:

A. Community-based nursing—NO, this is not the only correct option.

B. Community-oriented nursing—NO, this is not the only correct option.

C. Population-based nursing—NO, this is not the correct terminology.

D. Both A and B—YES, it refers to both.

Exhibit 1-1: Answer Details

Sometimes there is overlap. The key is to look at the focus of the care. If care is focused on the "health of the population," then it is community-oriented care. [(a) Doing routine health assessment is community-oriented nursing care.] If care is focused upon "illness care," then it is community-based nursing care. [(b) Providing medications for children with asthma, diabetes, or seizures is community-based nursing care.]

Exercise 1-8: *Fill-in*

Look at the table below, which lists the ANA Nursing and PHN Scope and Standards of Practice. Identify the similarities and differences between the two. Discuss the differences. Key differences are in bold and underlined. Please refer to the comments column for more detail.

Table 1-3: Comparison of ANA Nursing and PHN Scope and Standards of Practice

Nursing	Public Health Nursing	Notes
Standard 1—Assessment	Standard 1—Assessment	The focus of the public health nurse is on the diagnosis of health-related needs of *Populations* and priorities associated with these needs
Standard 2—Diagnosis	Standard 2—**Population** Diagnosis **and Priorities**	
Standard 3—Outcomes Identification	Standard 3—Outcomes Identification	
Standard 4—Planning	Standard 4—Planning	
Standard 5—Implementation	Standard 5—Implementation	
Standard 5a—Coordination of Care	Standard 5a—Coordination of Care	
Standard 5b—Health **Teaching** and Health Promotion	Standard 5b—Health **Education** and Health Promotion	
Standard 5c—Consultation	Standard 5c—Consultation	
Standard 5d—**Prescriptive Authority and Treatment**	Standard 5d—**Regulatory Activities**	

Table 1-3 *Continued*

Nursing	Public Health Nursing	Notes
Standard 6—Evaluation	Standard 6—Evaluation	The public health nurse provides health education *programs and services to populations.* This standard focuses on the application of and monitoring of public health laws and regulations
Standard 7—Quality of Practice	Standard 7—Quality of Practice	
Standard 8—Education	Standard 8—Education	
Standard 9—Professional Practice Evaluation	Standard 9—Professional Practice Evaluation	
Standard 10—Collegiality	Standard 10—Collegiality **and Professional Relationships**	
Standard 11—Collaboration		
Standard 12—Ethics	Standard 11—Collaboration	This standard focuses on the development of *"collegial partnerships while interacting with representatives of the population, organizations and health and human services professionals"* and contributing to the *"professional development of peers, students, colleagues, and others"* (ANA, 2007, p. 31)
Standard 13—Research	Standard 12—Ethics	
Standard 14—Resource Utilization	Standard 13—Research	
Standard 15—Leadership	Standard 14—Resource Utilization	
	Standard 15—Leadership	
	Standard 16—Advocacy	
		This standard focuses on the public health nurses' role to serve as an *"advocate to protect the health, safety and rights of the population"* (p. 40)

Source: ANA (2004, 2007).

Exhibit 1-2: Answer Details

The list of standards for Nursing Scope and Standards of Practice and for the Public Health Nursing (PHN) Scope and Standards of Practice look very similar except for a few words. But the descriptions of each standard for PHN show a focus on populations rather than on the individual.

Exercise 1-9: *Fill-in*

List the responsibilities of the community/public health nurse.

Responsibilities of community/public health nurses:

1. **Providing care to the ill and disabled in their homes, including teaching of caregivers**
2. **Maintaining healthful environments**
3. **Teaching about health promotion and prevention of disease and injury**
4. **Identifying those with inadequate standards of living and untreated illnesses and disabilities and referring them for services**
5. **Preventing and reporting neglect and abuse**
6. **Advocating for adequate standards of living and health care services**
7. **Collaborating to develop appropriate, adequate, acceptable health care services**
8. **Caring for oneself and participating in professional development activities**
9. **Ensuring quality nursing care and engaging in nursing research (Maurer & Smith, 2009, p. 15)**

Exercise 1-10: *Fill-in*

What are the core functions of public health?

1. **Assessment**
2. **Policy development**
3. **Assurance**

Exercise 1-11: *Fill-in*

Align the core public health function with the relevant essential public health service.

Table 1-4: Core Public Health Function

	Essential Public Health Services
Assessment	1. Monitor health status to identify and solve community health problems
Assessment	2. Diagnose and investigate health problems and health hazards in the community
Policy development	3. Inform, educate, and empower people about health issues

Table 1-4 *Continued*

	Essential Public Health Services
<u>Assurance</u>	4. Mobilize community partnerships and action to identify and solve health problems
<u>Policy development</u>	5. Develop policies and plans that support individual and community health efforts
<u>Policy development</u>	6. Enforce laws and regulations that protect health and ensure safety
<u>Assurance</u>	7. Link people to needed personal health services and ensure the provision of health care when otherwise unavailable
<u>Assurance</u>	8. Ensure competent public and personal health care workforce
<u>Assessment</u>	9. Evaluate effectiveness, accessibility, and quality of personal and population-based health services
<u>Policy development</u>	10. Research for new insights and innovative solutions to health problems

Exercise 1-12: *Select all that apply*

The principle of autonomy includes which of the following?

☒ **Protection of privacy**

❑ Paternalistic approach

☒ **Respect for the person**

☒ **Informed consent**

☒ **Fulfillment of client goals**

❑ Egalitarianism

Exercise 1-13: *Matching*

Match the term in column A with the definition in column B.

Column A	Column B
A. Autonomy	<u>**D.**</u> Concept that implies that some people are worthy to have a roof over their heads and others are not
B. Nonmaleficence	<u>**A.**</u> The condition of being independent and free to make your own decisions
C. Beneficence	<u>**B.**</u> To do no harm, an obligation to not intentionally or knowingly inflict harm
D. Distributive justice	<u>**C.**</u> Action taken for the benefit of others, to help prevent or remove harms or to improve the situation of others

Exercise 1-14: *Fill-in*

List factors that are determinants of health.

1. "Income and social status—higher income and social status are linked to better health. The greater the gap between the richest and the poorest people, the greater the differences in health.

2. Education—low education levels are linked with poor health, more stress, and lower self-confidence.

3. Physical environment—safe water and clean air, healthy workplaces, safe houses, communities, and roads all contribute to good health. Employment and working conditions—people in employment are healthier, particularly those who have more control over their working conditions.

4. Social support networks—greater support from families, friends, and communities is linked to better health. Culture, customs, and traditions, and the beliefs of the family and community all affect health.

5. Genetics—inheritance plays a part in determining life span, healthiness, and the likelihood of developing certain illnesses. Personal behavior and coping skills—balanced eating, keeping active, smoking, drinking, and how we deal with life's stresses and challenges all affect health.

6. Health services—access to and use of services that prevent and treat disease influence health.

7. Gender—"Men and women suffer from different types of diseases at different ages" (WHO, 2012a, p. 4).

Exercise 1-15: *Multiple-choice question*

One factor is primarily responsible for the differences in health care needs and health care outcomes among various countries. That factor is:

A. Economic development of the country—**YES, this is the primary factor.**

B. Political system of the country—NO, this is not the primary factor.

C. Social-cultural system of the country—NO, this is not the primary factor.

D. Religious faith of the country's main population—NO, this is not the primary factor.

Exercise 1-16: *Select all that apply*

What activities is a public health nurse likely to be involved in?

☒ **Collaborate with interdisciplinary teams to monitor and respond to health problems in population groups.**

☒ **Analyze health trends and risk factors of population groups to define priorities for targeted interventions.**

☒ **Collaborate with communities to develop targeted health promotion and disease prevention activities.**

☒ **Evaluate available health care services.**

☒ Provide health education, nursing care, case management, and primary care to vulnerable populations and high-risk groups.

☒ Participate in interdisciplinary programs that monitor, anticipate, and respond to public health problems.

☒ Appraise health trends, patterns, and risk factors of populations.

☒ Collaborate in development of public policy and targeted health promotion and disease prevention activities.

☒ Participate in efforts to disseminate information to promote health and reduce risk.

☒ Serve as an expert consultant on health matters.

☒ Appraise patterns and risk factors that present potential or actual environmental hazards and concerns.

Exercise 1-17: *Fill-in*

What is the value of core competencies …

1. To the profession?

    a. Serves as a mechanism to validate expertise

    b. Establishes standards and requisite skills

2. To the health care organization?

    a. Serves as a mechanism to develop job descriptions

    b. Serves as a mechanism to do performance and competency assessments/reviews

    c. Guides training programs and continuing education programs

3. To the public?

    a. Establishes a standard of professional practice that protects the public

    b. Provides a mechanism to measure outcomes

2

Epidemiology

"Epidemiology," says the instructor, "is very important in community/public health nursing. Remember, class, the focus of community-oriented nursing care is the health of *populations*. Therefore, a good understanding of epidemiology is essential if we are to have any success. So, let's start with a bit of history—a story to demonstrate how an understanding of epidemiology can have a significant impact upon the health of populations."

The class begins to learn about Dr. John Snow, the father of modern epidemiology, and his work in protecting the public's health. "John Snow," says the instructor, "is a very good example of the value of paying attention to emerging patterns (or trends) that are out of the norm." Anthony raises his hand. "Why is that important?" he asks. The instructor responds, "This observation and attention to detail can provide significant and meaningful insights into factors affecting health and what we can do to protect health. It is really about making sense of the data. Sometimes we have a lot of data but just didn't know how to interpret it. John Snow was the first to do this. Many of his principles we still use today."

To have the learners better understand the complexities of an epidemiological investigation such as the London Cholera Epidemic of 1854, the instructor provides additional materials to supplement the textbook readings.

 eResource 2-1: The instructor shows the class:
- UCLA Department of Epidemiology's presentation that provides a detailed overview about *The Life and Times of Dr. John Snow*: www.ph.ucla.edu/epi/snow.html
- UNC Gillings School of Global Public Health's case study: *John Snow Broad Street Pump Outbreak*: http://goo.gl/Uoeia

After completing the review of these materials, the instructor asks the class a series of questions:

Exercise 2-1: *Multiple-choice question*

John Snow's contribution to public health is:

      A. He is credited with stopping the cholera epidemic of 1854.

      B. He demonstrated the value of statistical analysis in public health.

      C. He created a system to ensure safe drinking water.

      D. He isolated the bacterium *Vibrio cholerae.*

      E. A, B

      F. A, B, and D

      G. All of the above

Exercise 2-2: *Multiple-choice question*

The best protection against contracting cholera is:

      A. Vaccination for cholera

      B. Avoiding people infected

      C. Avoiding contaminated food and water

      D. Avoiding undercooked food

Exercise 2-3: *Select all that apply*

Risk factors for contracting cholera include:

      ❑ Exposure to contaminated or untreated drinking water

      ❑ Droplet exposure to persons who have cholera

      ❑ Exposure to contaminated food

      ❑ Traveling to foreign countries

      ❑ Close contact with individuals who have not been immunized

The class discusses the pathophysiology of cholera and the importance of prompt and aggressive hydration and electrolyte replacement. "Remember, class, cholera is devastating, and if untreated can cause death within 24 hours. It can spread quickly. Therefore, it is important to identify the disease quickly and intervene promptly."

 eResource 2-2: To better understand the pathology of cholera and how it relates to osmosis, the instructor shows the class a brief lecture video, *Cholera and Osmosis:* http://youtu.be/9nRSzysJTyQ

Exercise 2-4: *Multiple-choice question*

In addition to fluid and electrolyte replacement, what other treatment should the patient receive?

      A. Antibiotic therapy

      B. Antimicrobial therapy

      C. Antidiarrheal therapy

      D. Anticholinergic therapy

      E. Antiviral therapy

Answers to this chapter begin on page 37.

The instructor asks the class, "Is there anything that can be done to prevent the spread of cholera among household contacts?"

Exercise 2-5: *Fill-in*
Describe measures to prevent transmission of cholera among household contacts.

_____

_____

_____

 eResource 2-3: To locate the answer to this question about cholera and preventive measures, Anthony opens Mobile MerckMedicus on his smartphone: [Pathway: Mobile MerckMedicus → Topics → enter "cholera" → select "cholera" → tap on menu in upper right corner to locate and select "prevention"]

The instructor explains to the class that in order for disease to occur, three things must be present. She asks the class to reflect upon the story of John Snow.

Exercise 2-6: *Fill-in*
Consider the cholera epidemic of 1854. Identify the host, agent, and environment within this outbreak.

      Host: _____

      Agent: _____

      Environment: _____

Before ending the class, the instructor asks the class to review some of the key epidemiologic terminology by playing a matching game.

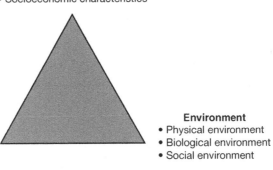

Figure 2-1: Epidemiological Triangle

Host
- Demographic characteristics
- Biological characteristics
- Socioeconomic characteristics

Agent
- Biological agents
- Physical agents
- Chemical agents
- Nutrient agents
- Mechanical agents
- Social agents

Environment
- Physical environment
- Biological environment
- Social environment

Answers to this chapter begin on page 37.

Exercise 2-7: *Matching*

Match the following terms with the correct definition.

A. Agent   _____ "A living intermediary that carries an agent from a reservoir to a susceptible host" (CDC, 2007)

B. Host   _____ "The ability of an infectious agent to cause severe disease, measured as the proportion of persons with the disease who become severely ill or die" (CDC, 2007)

C. Vector   _____ "A factor or form of energy whose presence or relative absence is essential for the occurrence of a disease or other adverse health outcome" (CDC, 2007)

D. Resistance   _____ "The ability of an agent to cause disease after infection, measured as the proportion of persons infected by an agent who then experience clinical disease" (CDC, 2007)

E. Nosocomial infections   _____ The capability of a body or an organism to defend itself against or fend off an infection

F. Reservoirs   _____ "A person or other living organism that is susceptible to or harbors an infectious agent under natural conditions" (CDC, 2007)

G. Virulence   _____ "The habitat in which an infectious agent normally lives, grows, and multiplies . . . ." (CDC, 2007)

H. Pathogenicity   _____ Hospital-acquired infections

I. Infectivity   _____ Ability to cause an immunologic response

J. Toxicity   _____ Ability of the host to remain free of illness despite exposure

K. Resistance   _____ Poisonous properties

L. Antigenicity   _____ Invasiveness

The next day, the instructor returns to the class discussion and asks the class to consider the mode of transmission of the infectious agent in the John Snow story. "In this situation, the organism was transmitted indirectly via contaminated water. Are there other ways that an infection can be transmitted?"

Answers to this chapter begin on page 37.

Exercise 2-8: *Fill-in*

List examples for mode of transmission:

Table 2-1:   Mode of Transmission

Mode of Transmission	Example
1. Airborne transmission	
2. Fecal-oral transmission	
3. Direct contact transmission	
4. Sexual contact transmission (this is a special instance of direct contact transmission)	
5. Direct inoculation transmission • Blood transfusion of contaminated blood • Use or accidental puncture by contaminated needles • Splash of contaminated body fluids on mucous membrane or a break in the skin	
6. Transplacental (vertical) Mother to fetus	
7. Animal or insect bite transmission	

"Historically," the instructor says, "communicable diseases have had a devastating effect—consider the high number of people in London who died as a result of cholera due to the contaminated water. What happened in London is considered an epidemic. You have heard the term pandemic. Can anyone explain what that is?"

Exercise 2-9: *Multiple-choice question*

The statement that most accurately describes a pandemic is:

A. Affecting or tending to affect an atypically large number of individuals within a population, community, or region at the same time (Merriam-Webster Incorporated, 2012)

B. An infectious outbreak spreading or capable of spreading rapidly to others (Merriam-Webster Incorporated, 2012)

C. An infectious disease transmissible by direct contact with an affected individual or the individual's discharges or by indirect means (Merriam-Webster Incorporated, 2012)

D. An outbreak of a disease that occurs over a wide geographic area and affects an exceptionally high proportion of the population (Merriam-Webster Incorporated, 2012)

The instructor asks the class, "Can anyone think of an example of a recent pandemic? I will give you a hint. It happened in 2009."

Answers to this chapter begin on page 37.

Exercise 2-10: *Fill-in*
What pandemic occurred in 2009?

_____

Exercise 2-11: *Multiple-choice question*
What was the mode of transmission for the 2009 pandemic?
   A. Airborne
   B. Vector
   C. Direct contact
   D. Fecal oral

The instructor moves the discussion to another communicable disease, Lyme disease. "Can anyone tell me the mode of transmission for Lyme disease?" she asks the class.

Exercise 2-12: *Multiple-choice question*
The mode of transmission for Lyme disease is
   A. Airborne transmission
   B. Vector transmission
   C. Direct contact transmission
   D. Fecal oral transmission

Exercise 2-13: *True or false*
Lyme disease is a concern only in the southeastern states.
   ❏ True
   ❏ False

Exercise 2-14: *Multiple-choice question*
The best way to remove an attached tick is:
   A. Use a hot match to burn it off
   B. Apply petroleum jelly
   C. Grasp the tick with tweezers close to the skin and pull
   D. All of the above

Exercise 2-15: *True or false*
A tick must be attached to a person's skin for more than 24 hours before it can transmit Lyme disease.
   ❏ True
   ❏ False

Answers to this chapter begin on page 37.

eResource 2-4: To learn more about Lyme disease and other vector-borne diseases, the class listens to the CDC's podcast on Vector-borne infection: http://goo.gl/z28pf

Unfolding Case Study #1 *Escherichia coli* Infection

Donna Parker is a new public health nurse working on the health surveillance team in the public health department. A report of a suspected outbreak of *E. coli* 0157 infection comes in. Twenty-nine people on the north side of the city developed bloody diarrhea after eating contaminated food. Another outbreak, affecting 11 people, was reported in the lower east side of the city. Two individuals were hospitalized with hemorrhagic colitis and thrombotic thrombocytopenic purpura.

Donna remembers the recent training she had when first starting at the public health department. She remembers that for disease to occur, three things must be present: host, agent, and environment.

In addition, she recalls the key components of public health surveillance.

Exercise 2-16: *Fill-in*
What is surveillance?

_____

_____

_____

Exercise 2-17: *Fill-in*
What is the purpose of surveillance?

_____

_____

_____

 eResource 2-5: As Donna prepares to participate in the investigation, she takes the opportunity to review some of the materials from her recent training:
- Video entitled *E. Coli 0157* from the Discovery Channel [Pathway: http://goo.gl/YRern. Using the scroll on the "Killer Outbreaks Videos" playlist button, select "*E. coli* 0157"]
- Video entitled *Foodborne Illness: A Handy Overview* by Barbara Mahon, MD, MPH: http://goo.gl/YRjYX

■ *Shiga Toxin-Producing* Escherichia Coli *Infections: What Clinicians Need to Know* by Rajal Mody, MD, MPH, and Phillip I. Tarr, MD
  ■ Audio presentation: http://goo.gl/wWGxz
  ■ Handouts: http://goo.gl/dJzUf

Even though she has reviewed the materials, Donna also wants to make sure that she is prepared to answer questions as she conducts interviews with people in the community. She makes sure that she has information readily available on her mobile device for quick access so she can answer any questions that arise. She particularly anticipates that people will have specific questions regarding the bacteria, any long-term effects, risk factors, and steps the government will take.

 eResource 2-6: Donna accesses the following resources on her smartphone in preparation for questions from members of the community:
  ■ FoodSafety.gov [Pathway: www.foodsafety.gov → select "food poisoning" → select "*E. coli*" and review related sections]
  ■ Mobile MerckMedicus [Pathway: MerckMedicus → select "Topics" → enter "*E. coli*" → select "*Escherichia coli* infection" → select "0157/H7 infection"]

As the investigation progresses, it is discovered that these two cases are linked with 38 others in the same community.

Exercise 2-18: *Multiple-choice question*
Which of the following terms indicates the number or proportion of persons in a population who have a disease at a given point in time?
  A. Sensitivity
  B. Prevalence
  C. Negative predictive value
  D. None of the above

Exercise 2-19: *Matching*
Match the following epidemiology terms with the appropriate definition.

A. Incidence   _____ The number or proportion of cases or events or conditions in a given population

B. Prevalence   _____ The relative size of two quantities, calculated by dividing one quantity by the other

C. Rate   _____ Disease; any departure from a state of physiological or psychological health and well-being

D. Ratio   _____ The frequency with which an event, such as a new case of illness, occurs in a population over a period of time

Answers to this chapter begin on page 37.

E. Morbidity   _____ The frequency of occurrence of death among a
defined population during a specified time interval

F. Mortality rate   _____ The frequency with which an event occurs in a
defined population during a specified period divided
by population

The Public Health Surveillance Team goes out to interview all of the individuals affected to identify any commonalities. Donna knows that this type of data collection is called public health surveillance.

Donna recalls that the World Health Organization defines public health surveillance as the "continuous, systematic collection, analysis and interpretation of health-related data needed for the planning, implementation, and evaluation of public health practice" (2012b, p. 1). Donna understands that this process involves several activities.

Exercise 2-20: *Multiple-choice question*
Public health surveillance involves which of the following activities?
> A. Serving as a late warning system for public health concerns
> B. Documentation of the impact of an intervention
> C. Marketing efforts to highlight progress toward specified goals
> D. Monitoring and clarifying the pathogenicity of health problems

Exercise 2-21: *Multiple-choice question*
The constant presence of a disease or infectious agent within a given geographic area or population group is referred to as:
> A. Epidemic
> B. Pandemic
> C. Endemic
> D. Contagion

Donna also recalls that there are a variety of surveillance systems that collect reportable data.

Exercise 2-22: *Matching*
Match the following terms with the correct definition.

A. Universal case reporting   _____ A surveillance system in which reports
are obtained from certain facilities or
populations

B. Sentinel surveillance   _____ A surveillance system in which the
reports of cases come from clinical
laboratories instead of health care
practitioners or hospitals

Answers to this chapter begin on page 37.

C. Laboratory-based reporting   _____ A surveillance system in which all cases of a disease are supposed to be reported

D. Zoonotic disease surveillance   _____ A surveillance method that uses clinical information about disease signs and symptoms, before a diagnosis is made

E. Syndromic surveillance   _____ Surveillance of diseases found in animals that can be transmitted to humans and often involves a system for detecting infected animals (Anderson, 2008)

Donna remembers that there are two main types of surveillance: active and passive.

Exercise 2-23: *Multiple-choice question*

Which statement below best describes passive surveillance?

        A. Passive surveillance is the action of receiving and collecting health data undertaken by public health authorities.

        B. Passive surveillance is health departments receiving information regarding legally reportable conditions.

        C. Passive surveillance is public health department outreach activities to assimilate health data.

        D. Passive surveillance involves field deployment to clinics, hospitals, and clinical laboratories.

Donna also remembers that surveillance involves a systematic approach that collects data and includes the same additional activities. She remembers that during orientation the course facilitator showed the class a list of activities and asked, "Which of these activities would be considered as part of public health surveillance?"

Exercise 2-24: *Select all that apply*

Which of the following activities would be included in public health surveillance?

    ❑ Detecting outbreaks and threats

    ❑ Proactively contacting individuals in the community

    ❑ Finding cases for intervention

    ❑ Monitoring trends

    ❑ Making routine site visits to all health care facilities

    ❑ Directing interventions

    ❑ Evaluating interventions

    ❑ Generating hypotheses

The epidemiologic investigation linked these 2 cases and 38 others in the same community to a local restaurant that had offered a salad bar with Romaine lettuce

Answers to this chapter begin on page 37.

being the suspected vehicle of transmission. The source of the infection was determined to be improper handling of the food during transport to the restaurant. Through this investigative process, all affected packages of Romaine lettuce were removed and destroyed to prevent additional infection.

Donna reflects on this experience and realizes that this process is only one aspect of public health surveillance and the information obtained from this and other ongoing surveillance provide data that can inform and guide provision of public health actions and interventions.

Exercise 2-25: *Select all that apply*
Which of the following are public health actions and interventions that could be obtained from public health surveillance?
    A. Prophylaxis
    B. Education
    C. Early identification of problems
    D. Prevention and control
    E. Health care cost containment

Now that the outbreak has been contained, the surveillance team uses the public's heightened awareness of food safety issues as an opportunity to educate, and plans a food safety education program.

Unfolding Case Study #2   *Salmonella* Outbreak

Anita McCall is a school nurse for an elementary school in a rural community. She notices that there are an increased number of students coming to her office complaining of fever, nausea, vomiting, and abdominal cramps. She makes arrangements for the parents of the more severely affected children to come to the school to take the children home or to the family physician. Six children had to go home. At least five other children came to her office complaining of milder symptoms, but Anita suspects that there may be more.

Exercise 2-26: *Multiple-choice question*
Sending the more severely affected children home meets which of the following public health actions and interventions warranted when there is a suspected outbreak?
    A. Prophylaxis
    B. Education
    C. Prevention and control
    D. Early identification of problems

The following day, a mother calls Anita and tells her that her son, Ryan, was diagnosed as having *Salmonella* poisoning. Anita thinks about all of the children that came to her office yesterday. The more she thinks about it, the more she believes

Answers to this chapter begin on page 37.

that all the children were presenting the same symptoms as Ryan and begins to suspect that there may be a problem in the school cafeteria.

 eResource 2-7: Anita consults the Massachusetts Department of Public Health Guidelines regarding *Salmonella* outbreak management: http://goo.gl/oJQ6p

Anita notifies the school principal and together they prepare to alert the school faculty and staff as well as the parents. In addition, as required by the Massachusetts Department of Public Health, Anita notifies the local health department.

 eResource 2-8: In addition, Anita consults the following resources to learn more about outbreak investigations and reportable diseases:
- System (NNDSS): wwwn.cdc.gov/nndss/
- Outbreak Investigations: http://goo.gl/S3zvU

Anita also wants to update her knowledge about salmonellosis and treatment so she can prepare a memo to send out to the school teachers, staff, and parents. She looks for information from the Centers for Disease Control and Prevention (CDC) and the local public health department and prepares an information packet for the school teachers, staff, and parents.

 eResource 2-9: Anita uses the following to prepare handouts information:
- FoodSafety.gov [Pathway: www.foodsafety.gov → select "food poisoning" → select "*Salmonella*" and review related sections]
- Patient Handouts about salmonellosis food poisoning from Merck Medicus: [Pathway: www.merckmedicus.com → select "Patient Handouts" → enter "*Salmonella*" into the search field and select desired handout]

Following Anita's notification of the local health department, Veronica Smith, the public health nurse who works on the surveillance team, comes to the school to assess and investigate the outbreak. Veronica knows that she needs to first determine if there really is an outbreak, so she reflects upon what factors she must consider.

Exercise 2-27: *Select all that apply*
To determine if an outbreak exists, which of the following factors must be considered?
- ❏ Increased number of cases for a given time, place, and population
- ❏ More severe disease presentation
- ❏ Usual exposure routes to pathogens
- ❏ Presenting disease is common for a given area (disease that is unusual for a given area)
- ❏ Outbreaks with zoonotic and human component
- ❏ Typical strains or variants of organisms (unusual strains or variants of organisms)

Answers to this chapter begin on page 37.

Anita tells Veronica that she thinks that the outbreak may be related to some caf-eteria food, but she has not been able to identify any common food item that all children may have ingested. Veronica tells Anita that until they know more, it is a good idea to close the cafeteria and have children, faculty, and staff bring their own lunches from home for the time being. She goes on to tell Anita that the first thing she plans to do is conduct interviews and collect more information to determine if there actually is an outbreak. "We also need to perform descriptive epidemiology and develop a line listing."

Warren looks confused. "What's that?"

Exercise 2-28: *Fill-in*

What is descriptive epidemiology and what is a line listing?

_____

_____

_____

Veronica tells Anita, "As you know, the most important step when an outbreak is suspected is to implement control and prevention measures. You did a nice job of getting the affected students out of the school, but we need to do more."

Exercise 2-29: *Select all that apply*

Which of the following are control and prevention measures?

- ❑ Removing the ill food handler
- ❑ Recalling contaminated food product
- ❑ Analyzing incident retrospectively
- ❑ Closing the restaurant or manufacturing plant
- ❑ Implementing new protective policies
- ❑ Cleaning up contamination
- ❑ Providing prophylaxis to exposed population
- ❑ Communication

Veronica conducts interviews and completes the line listing. She determines that while all the children affected by the *Salmonella* outbreak were in different classes and ate different food, they share a common recess period. Through interviewing the children, Veronica discovers that a young boy, Ronnie, had brought a small turtle he had found in a local pond to school in his pocket and was showing it to the other children and letting them handle the turtle during recess. Veronica inter-views Ronnie and verifies that the turtle is indeed the vector.

 eResource 2-10: Anita prepares updated information to disseminate.
- Pet turtles and *Salmonella*: http://youtu.be/tvZiIeTZ0vE
- CDC report on *Multistate Outbreaks of Human* Salmonella *Infections Linked to Small Turtles*: http://goo.gl/Nw2tm
- CDC podcast, *The Trouble with Turtles*: http://goo.gl/CXaFM

Answers to this chapter begin on page 37.

As they wrap up the report, Veronica tells Anita about a previous *Salmonella* outbreak that occurred in June of last year. "There was a widespread report of people getting sick, and we suspected that it was due to contaminated tomatoes. What do you think was our first step?"

Exercise 2-30: *Fill-in*
After determining that the source of the contamination was tomatoes, what should Veronica and the surveillance team have done next?

_____

_____

_____

Veronica tells Anita, "We did a large number of interviews and that led to the hypothesis that it was the tomatoes—so we issued a tomato alert. People stopped eating tomatoes. But the incidence of the *Salmonella* did not decrease. What do you think we had to do next?"

Exercise 2-31: *Fill-in*
What is the next step?

_____

_____

_____

The key points here are:
- Communication is essential
- Maintain communication throughout investigation
- Implement control measures early and typically before the investigation is fully completed (e.g., tomato alert)
- Focus is to control the outbreak and prevent additional spread—ultimate goal

Answers to this chapter begin on page 37.

Answers

Exercise 2-1: *Multiple-choice question*

John Snow's contribution to public health is:

A. He is credited with stopping the cholera epidemic of 1854—YES, this is correct.

B. He demonstrated the value of statistical analysis in public health—YES, this is correct.

C. He created a system to ensure safe drinking water—NO

D. He isolated the bacterium *Vibrio cholerae*—NO

E. A, B—YES, both are correct.

F. A, B, and D—NO, not D

G. All of the above—NO, not C and D

Exercise 2-2: *Multiple-choice question*

The best protection against contracting cholera is:

A. Vaccination for cholera—NO, this is not possible.

B. Avoiding people infected—NO, this is not the transmission

C. Avoiding contaminated food and water—YES

D. Avoiding undercooked food—NO, it is contaminated.

Exercise 2-3: *Select all that apply*

Risk factors for contracting cholera include:

☒ **Exposure to contaminated or untreated drinking water—YES**

❑ Droplet exposure to persons who have cholera—NO, wrong transmission

☒ **Exposure to contaminated food—YES**

❑ Traveling to foreign countries—NO, this in itself is not a risk.

❑ Close contact with individual who have not been immunized—NO

Exercise 2-4: *Multiple-choice question*

In addition to fluid and electrolyte replacement, what other treatment should the patient receive?

A. Antibiotic therapy—NO, it is a microbe.

B. Antimicrobial therapy—YES

C. Antidiarrheal therapy—NO, it is a microbe.

D. Anticholinergic therapy—NO, it is a microbe.

E. Antiviral therapy—NO, it is a microbe.

Exercise 2-5: *Fill-in*

Describe measures to prevent transmission of cholera among household contacts.

Human waste must be properly disposed of; water supplies need to be purified (boiled or chlorinated); fish and vegetables need to be cooked thoroughly.

Exhibit 2-1: Answer Details

For prevention and control of cholera, among household members, prompt prophylaxis medication administration is indicated:

- Doxycycline 100 mg orally every 12 hours in adults

- TMP-SMX can be used for prophylaxis in children <9 years

Exercise 2-6: *Fill-in*

Consider the cholera epidemic of 1854. Identify the host, agent, and environment within this outbreak.

Host: **People of London's SoHo District**

Agent: **The bacterium *Vibrio cholerae***

Environment: **Poor sanitation conditions; contaminated water from the Broad Street Pump**

Exercise 2-7: *Matching*

Match the following terms with the correct definition.

A. Agent	**C**	"A living intermediary that carries an agent from a reservoir to a susceptible host" (CDC, 2007)
B. Host	**G**	"The ability of an infectious agent to cause severe disease, measured as the proportion of persons with the disease who become severely ill or die" (CDC, 2007)
C. Vector	**A**	"A factor or form of energy whose presence or relative absence is essential for the occurrence of a disease or other adverse health outcome" (CDC, 2007)
D. Resistance	**H**	"The ability of an agent to cause disease after infection, measured as the proportion of persons infected by an agent who then experience clinical disease" (CDC, 2007)
E. Nosocomial infections	**K**	The capability of a body or an organism to defend itself against or fend off an infection
F. Reservoirs	**B**	"A person or other living organism that is susceptible to or harbors an infectious agent under natural conditions" (CDC, 2007)
G. Virulence	**F**	"The habitat in which an infectious agent normally lives, grows, and multiplies. . . ." (CDC, 2007)

H. Pathogenicity ___**E**__ Hospital-acquired infections

I. Infectivity ___**L**__ Ability to cause an immunologic response

J. Toxicity ___**K**__ Ability of the host to remain free of illness despite exposure

K. Resistance ___**J**__ Poisonous properties

L. Antigenicity ___**I**__ Invasiveness

Exercise 2-8: *Fill-in*

List examples for mode of transmission:

Table 2-2: Mode of Transmission

Mode of Transmission	Example
1. Airborne transmission	Anthrax, influenza, pneumonia
2. Fecal-oral transmission	*Salmonella*
3. Direct contact transmission	Skin to skin contact
4. Sexual contact transmission (this is a special instance of direct contact transmission)	STDs, HIV/AIDS, hepatitis
5. Direct inoculation transmission • Blood transfusion of contaminated blood • Use or accidental puncture by contaminated needles • Splash of contaminated body fluids on mucous membrane or a break in the skin	HIV/AIDS, hepatitis
6. Trans-placental (vertical) Mother to fetus	Congenital rubella, congenital varicella, cytomegalovirus inclusion disease, HIV
7. Animal or insect bite transmission	Malaria, rabies, Lyme disease

Exercise 2-9: *Multiple-choice question*

The statement that most accurately describes a pandemic is:

A. Affecting or tending to affect an atypically large number of individuals within a population, community, or region at the same time (Merriam-Webster Incorporated, 2012)—NO, this is not the correct definition.

B. An infectious outbreak spreading or capable of spreading rapidly to others (Merriam-Webster Incorporated, 2012)—NO, this is not the correct definition.

C. An infectious disease transmissible by direct contact with an affected individual or the individual's discharges or by indirect means (Merriam-Webster Incorporated, 2012)—NO, this is not the correct definition.

D. **An outbreak of a disease that occurs over a wide geographic area and affects an exceptionally high proportion of the population (Merriam-Webster Incorporated, 2012)—YES**

Exercise 2-10: *Fill-in*

What pandemic occurred in 2009?

Pandemic (H1N1) in 2009, also known as the swine flu pandemic.

Exercise 2-11: *Multiple-choice question*

What was the mode of transmission for the 2009 pandemic?

A. Airborne—YES

B. Vector—NO, this is not the transmission.

C. Direct contact—NO, this is not the transmission.

D. Fecal oral—NO, this is not the transmission.

Exercise 2-12: *Multiple-choice question*

The mode of transmission for Lyme disease is:

A. Airborne transmission—NO, this is not the transmission.

B. Vector transmission—YES

C. Direct contact transmission—NO, this is not the transmission.

D. Fecal oral transmission—NO, this is not the transmission.

Exercise 2-13: *True or false*

Lyme disease is a concern only in the southeastern states.

❑ True

☒ **False—YES**

Exercise 2-14: *Multiple-choice question*

The best way to remove an attached tick is:

A. Use a hot match to burn it off—NO, this is dangerous.

B. Apply petroleum jelly—NO, this is not effective.

C. Grasp the tick with tweezers close to the skin and pull—YES

D. All of the above—NO

Exercise 2-15: *True or false*

A tick must be attached to a person's skin for more than 24 hours before it can transmit Lyme disease.

☒ **True—YES**

❑ False

Exhibit 2-2: Answer Details

To learn more about Lyme disease, go to: www.cdc.gov/lyme.

Exercise 2-16: *Fill-in*

What is surveillance?

"**Public health surveillance is the ongoing, systematic collection, analysis, and interpretation of data that is then disseminated to those responsible for preventing diseases and other health conditions. The data allow managers to respond quickly to a population's health needs. This information is also essential for ministries of health, ministries of finance, and donors to monitor how well people are served. Surveillance enables decision makers to lead and manage effectively**" (Disease Control Priorities Project, 2008, p. 1).

Exercise 2-17: *Fill-in*

What is the purpose of surveillance?

Surveillance tells us where the problems are, who is affected, and where the programmatic and prevention activities should be directed. "Public health surveillance provides real-time, early warning information to decision makers about health problems that need to be addressed in a particular population. It is a critical tool to prevent outbreaks of diseases and develop appropriate, rapid responses when diseases begin to spread" (Disease Control Priorities Project, 2008, p. 1).

Exercise 2-18: *Multiple-choice question*

Which of the following terms indicates the number or proportion of persons in a population who have a disease at a given point in time?

A. Sensitivity—NO, this is not the term.

B. Prevalence—YES

C. Negative predictive value—NO, this is not the proper term.

D. None of the above—NO

Exercise 2-19: *Matching*

Match the following epidemiology terms with the appropriate definition.

A. Incidence	__**A**__	The number or proportion of cases or events or conditions in a given population
B. Prevalence	__**D**__	The relative size of two quantities, calculated by dividing one quantity by the other
C. Rate	__**E**__	Disease; any departure from a state of physiological or psychological health and well-being
D. Ratio	__**A**__	The frequency with which an event, such as a new case of illness, occurs in a population over a period of time
E. Morbidity	__**F**__	The frequency of occurrence of death among a defined population during a specified time interval

F. Mortality rate   **__B__** The frequency with which an event occurs in a defined population during a specified period divided by population

Exercise 2-20: *Multiple-choice questions*
Public health surveillance involves which of the following activities?
A. Serving as a late warning system for public health concerns—NO, this is too late.
B. Documentation of the impact of an intervention—YES, this is an appropriate activity.
C. Marketing efforts to highlight progress toward specified goals—NO
D. Monitoring and clarifying the pathogenicity of health problems—NO

Exhibit 2-3: Answer Details

Public health surveillance can:

- Serve as an *early warning system* for impending public health emergencies

- Document the impact of an intervention

- Track progress toward specified goals

- Monitor and clarify the epidemiology of health problems, to allow priorities to be set and to inform public health policy and strategies

Source: World Health Organization (2012b).

Exercise 2-21: *Multiple-choice question*
The constant presence of a disease or infectious agent within a given geographic area or population group is referred to as:
A. Epidemic—NO, this is the wrong term.
B. Pandemic—NO, this is the wrong term.
C. Endemic—YES
D. Contagion—NO, this is the wrong term.

Exercise 2-22: *Matching*
Match the following terms with the correct definition.

A. Universal case reporting   **__A__** A surveillance system in which reports are obtained from certain facilities or populations

B. Sentinel surveillance   **__C__** A surveillance system in which the reports of cases come from clinical laboratories instead of health care practitioners or hospitals

C. Laboratory-based reporting

D. Zoonotic disease surveillance

E. Syndromic surveillance

___A___ A surveillance system in which all cases of a disease are supposed to be reported

___E___ A surveillance method that uses clinical information about disease signs and symptoms, before a diagnosis is made

___D___ Surveillance of diseases found in animals that can be transmitted to humans and often involves a system for detecting infected animals (Anderson, 2008)

Exercise 2-23: *Multiple-choice question*

What statement below best describes passive surveillance?

A. Passive surveillance is the action of receiving and collecting health data undertaken by public health authorities—NO

B. Passive surveillance is health departments receiving information regarding legally reportable conditions—YES

C. Passive surveillance is public health department outreach activities to assimilate health data—NO

D. Passive surveillance involves field deployment to clinics, hospitals, and clinical laboratories—NO

Exercise 2-24: *Select all that apply*

Which of the following activities would be included in public health surveillance?

☒ **Detecting outbreaks and threats**

☐ Proactively contacting individuals in the community

☒ **Finding cases for intervention**

☒ **Monitoring trends**

☐ Making routine site visits to all health care facilities

☒ **Directing interventions**

☒ **Evaluating interventions**

☒ **Generating hypotheses**

Exercise 2-25: *Select all that apply*

Which of the following are public health actions and interventions that could be obtained from public health surveillance?

A. **Prophylaxis (mass immunizations to combat epidemic or pandemic or bioterrorism)—YES, this is an activity for surveillance.**

B. **Education (education of public, e.g., stay away from crowds in public places)— YES, this is an activity.**

C. Early identification of problems (this is part of surveillance and provides the information that *"guides and informs"* public health actions and interventions)—NO

D. **Prevention and control (knowing what the problem is; can help with focused efforts to prevent further spread)—YES, this is an activity**.

E. Health care cost containment (this is a possible outcome of the public health actions and interventions)—NO

Exercise 2-26: *Multiple-choice question*

Sending the more severely affected children home meets which of the following public health actions and interventions warranted when there is a suspected outbreak?

A. Prophylaxis—NO, this is already too late.

B. Education—NO, this is already too late.

C. **Prevention and control—YES, this is the intervention.**

D. Early identification of problems—NO, this is already too late.

Exercise 2-27: *Select all that apply*

To determine if an outbreak exists, which of the following factors must be considered?

☒ **Increased number of cases for a given time, place, and population—YES**

☒ **More severe disease presentation—YES**

☒ **Usual exposure routes to pathogens—YES**

❑ Presenting disease is common for a given area (disease that is unusual for a given area)—NO, this is restrictive.

☒ **Outbreaks with zoonotic and human component—YES**

❑ Typical strains or variants of organisms (unusual strains or variants of organisms)—NO, this is not typical.

Exercise 2-28: *Fill-in*

What is descriptive epidemiology and what is a line listing?

In the disease investigation process, performing descriptive epidemiology involves describing person, place, and time of the onset of signs and symptoms (S/S) and detailed description of the S/S. The line listing is a chronological listing of the events surrounding the outbreak, identifying each person affected, S/S, where he or she was (or likely was) prior to the onset of S/S.

Exercise 2-29: *Select all that apply*

Which of the following are control and prevention measures?

☒ **Removing the ill food handler**

☒ **Recalling contaminated food product**

❑ Analyzing incident retrospectively

☒ **Closing the restaurant or manufacturing plant**

❑ Implementing new protective policies

☒ Cleaning up contamination

☒ Providing prophylaxis to exposed population

☒ Communication

Exercise 2-30: *Fill-in*

After determining that the source of contamination was tomatoes, what should Veronica and the surveillance team have done next?

Implement control and prevention measures ASAP

- **Should be done ASAP and as information is obtained, there should be communication to the public to prevent and control the spread. This is:**
  - **Source intervention**
  - **Interruption of transmission route**
  - **Disrupt the natural history of the disease**
- **Examples: issuing a tomato recall, getting this produce off the store shelves, alerting the public not to eat tomatoes, and so forth**

Exercise 2-31: *Fill-in*

What is the next step?

Re-examine the hypothesis.

Re-interview the people to find out any other commonality between the individuals affected. In this instance, the investigators found that in addition to eating a lot of tomatoes, the affected individuals also ate jalapeno peppers. Further investigation determined that the source was the jalapeno peppers. A jalapeno alert was issued and the cases of *Salmonella* dropped.

The key points here are:

- **Communication is essential**
- **Maintain communication throughout investigation**
- **Implement control measures early and typically before the investigation is fully completed (e.g., tomato alert)**

Focus is to control the outbreak and prevent additional spread—the ultimate goal.

3

Communicable Diseases

Unfolding Case Study #1 ▒ Flu Immunization Program

The class learns that participating in the monitoring of health trends and patterns, including communicable diseases such as the flu, is an essential role for the public health nurse. "Remember, class," said the instructor, "the goal is to *protect the health* of the population and the nurse is uniquely positioned to work closely with the community and provide not only essential health education, but also to assist in implementation of protective measures such as immunization."

To highlight the importance of this, the instructor provides a brief overview of how epidemics and pandemics have historically caused significant mortality and morbidity worldwide. Contemporary public health methods have done much to help contain communicable diseases and avoid the even higher death rates experienced in the past. She tells them that while there have been outbreaks recently, "the flu pandemic of 1918 to 1919 was the deadliest in modern history, infected an estimated 500 million people worldwide—about one-third of the planet's population at the time—and killed an estimated 20 million to 50 million victims. More than 25 percent of the U.S. population became sick, and some 675,000 Americans died during the pandemic" (1918 Flu Pandemic, 2012, p. 1).

 eResource 3-1: To understand the impact of the 1918 flu pandemic, the class views two videos:
- ▒ *We Heard the Bells: The Influenza of 1918:*
  http://youtu.be/XbEefT_M6xY
- ▒ *Hospitals "Full-Up": The 1918 Influenza Pandemic:*
  youtu.be/tpzxNoLZx0w

The instructor tells the class that while the flu pandemic affected a lot of people, there are certain populations that are particularly vulnerable and therefore focused community outreach and education efforts are essential. She shows a third video to underscore this point.

 eResource 3-2: *Remembering the 1918 Flu Epidemic:*
http://youtu.be/pNP9KwFMU6Y

Exercise 3-1: *Fill-in*

Following the video presentations, the instructor asks the following questions:

1. What factors contributed to the spread of the flu in 1918?

_____

_____

2. What factors or conditions put a person at risk for contracting the flu?

_____

_____

3. What is the most effective way to protect against the flu?

_____

_____

Exercise 3-2: *True or false*

A person who gets the flu shot is immediately protected against the flu.

    A. True

    B. False

The instructor continues the lecture by highlighting how important it is that all health care providers fully understand all vaccinations—who needs to have them—and that they are aware of *all possible contraindications and precautions* for health conditions that might preclude a particular vaccine. "The key," the instructor stresses, "is for the health care provider to be knowledgeable. Frequently misunderstandings and misconceptions lead to missed opportunities to protect the public's health." The instructor provides students with a handout that highlights this information.

(e)   **eResource 3-3:** The instructor locates the State of Minnesota's Guidelines and shares these with the class: http://goo.gl/ak8jC

Exercise 3-3: *Select all that apply*

In regard to routine immunizations, which of the following is not an appropriate procedure for the health care provider to follow?

    ❑ Always administer vaccines as indicated on the immunization schedule

    ❑ Avoid missing opportunities to vaccinate

    ❑ Avoid administering immunizations to pregnant women

    ❑ Screen patients each time prior to vaccinating

Answers to this chapter begin on page 69.

Exercise 3-4: *Select all that apply*

Which of the following criteria is a contraindication for administering the diphtheria, tetanus, pertussis (DTaP) vaccine?

- ❏ Temperature of 104°F following previous administration of the DTP or DTaP vaccine
- ❏ Family history of seizures
- ❏ Encephalopathy of unknown etiology within 7 days following previous administration of the DTP or DTaP vaccine
- ❏ Family history of sudden infant death syndrome
- ❏ Family history of an adverse event after DTP or DTaP administration
- ❏ Immunodeficient family member or household contact

The instructor tells the class that as part of their clinical experience, they will all be able to participate in Minneapolis' citywide seasonal flu immunization program, so this week's lecture will provide an important overview to prepare the students for this experience.

The instructor tells the students that an important role of the Centers for Disease Control and Prevention (CDC) is to monitor outbreaks—which happen every year—and put into place measures to protect the public's health. The "flu season" begins in mid-to-late fall, peaks in January or February, and runs until spring. Every year "more than 200,000 Americans are hospitalized for flu-related complications, and over the past three decades, there have been some 3,000 to 49,000 flu-related deaths in the U.S. annually" (CDC, 2011a, p. 1).

Trevor raises his hand and asks, "How do we know how severe the flu season will be?" The instructor answers, "The flu is unpredictable and how severe it is varies from season to season. The severity is affected by how well we identify the flu viruses that are spreading and then make a vaccine that is matched to flu viruses that are causing illness."

Exercise 3-5: *Multiple-choice question*

Other factors affecting the severity of the flu season include all of the following except:

- A. How much flu vaccine is available
- B. Route along which the vaccine is administered
- C. When the flu vaccine is available
- D. How many people get vaccinated

The instructor tells the class, "There are many activities in which the public health nurse can become involved to help prevent widespread influenza infection. Let's make a list. What are some of these activities that can take place prior to the flu season to prepare the public?" The class begins to buzz as the students talk among themselves.

Answers to this chapter begin on page 69.

Exercise 3-6: *Multiple-choice question*

Which of the following activities/strategies can be utilized to prevent or minimize widespread influenza infection?

    A. Conduct community outreach program

    B. Offer flu shot clinics

    C. Teach regarding proper hand washing

    D. Take antiviral medications as prescribed by the physician

    E. All of the above

    F. A, B, and C

The instructor reminds the students that surveillance is an important component during the flu season. Reportable diseases are monitored closely and reported weekly to ensure timely and appropriate response. "There are a variety of resources available that can help us see how the flu season is unfolding."

 eResource 3-4:
■ Weekly U.S. Map: Influenza Summary Update:
www.cdc.gov/flu/weekly/usmap.htm
■ Weekly Influenza Surveillance Report: http://goo.gl/Kdgwn

The instructor asks the class, "Is everyone at the same risk level for getting the flu?"

Exercise 3-7: *Select all that apply*

Which of the following group(s) is (are) particularly vulnerable to flu-related complications?

    ❑ Young children

    ❑ Nursing babies

    ❑ People over age 65

    ❑ Adolescents

    ❑ Pregnant women

    ❑ Recent immigrants

    ❑ People with asthma

    ❑ People with diabetes

The instructor goes on to tell the class, "Remember, earlier we looked at a document that provided an overview of precautions and contraindications for administering immunizations. Even though we know that some people are at higher risk, we also need to know if there are any other factors that must be considered prior to administration of the flu vaccine. It is the responsibility of the health care provider to keep up-to-date with this information. A good source is the CDC and the World Health Organization (WHO)."

Answers to this chapter begin on page 69.

eResource 3-5:
- CDC Vaccine Information: www.cdc.gov/vaccines/default.htm
- WHO: www.who.int/immunization/policy/Immunization_routine_
  table1.pdf

Exercise 3-8: *Multiple-choice question*
Which of the following are contraindications for administering the influenza "live" attenuated (LAIV) vaccine?

    A. Pregnant or breastfeeding family member or household contact

    B. Breastfeeding

    C. Children who are on aspirin therapy

    D. Health care workers that care for patients in protective isolation

    E. Contacts of persons with chronic medical conditions

The class reviews key terminology associated with communicable diseases. The instructor asks a series of questions to determine the students' understanding.

Exercise 3-9: *Multiple-choice question*
Which of the following definitions from the CDC (2007) accurately describes passive immunity?

    A. "Resistance developed in response to an antigen (i.e., an infecting agent or vaccine), usually characterized by the presence of antibody produced by the host"

    B. "The resistance to an infectious agent of an entire group or community as a result of a substantial proportion of the population being immune to the agent"

    C. "Immunity conferred by an antibody produced in another host"

Exercise 3-10: *Multiple-choice question*
Which would be considered a host in the chain of infection?

    A. Human

    B. Excessive heat

    C. Overcrowding

    D. *Escherichia coli*

Exercise 3-11: *Multiple-choice question*
An individual acquires artificial immunity by:

    A. Being vaccinated

    B. Previous infection with the disease

    C. Previous exposure to the disease

    D. From the body's antigen-antibody response to infection

    E. Having a compromised immune system

Answers to this chapter begin on page 69.

To learn more about epidemiology and immunization, the class is instructed to take the opportunity to attend the CDC's free, on-demand training via the Training and Continuing Education Online System and to review available materials.

 eResource 3-6:
  ■ *Epidemiology & Prevention of Vaccine-Preventable Diseases*: www2a.cdc.gov/TCEOnline
  ■ Resources: http://goo.gl/lzxgN

Susan and Ted are two students participating in a flu clinic at a community center in the northeast section of the city. They are looking forward to the experience but want to make sure that they are properly prepared to participate in the clinic.

 eResource 3-7: Prior to attending the flu clinic, they review materials:
  ■ CDC's Seasonal Influenza (Flu) information: www.cdc.gov/flu/index.htm
  ■ Screening Questionnaire: www.immunize.org/catg.d/p4066.pdf
  ■ CDC Publications: http://goo.gl/lzxgN

When the students arrive at the flu clinic, the nurse in charge provides an orientation to the group. She assigns the students in pairs to each station. She reminds the students that for each client, they need to complete the screening process prior to administering the flu shot. Ted and Susan are assigned to work as a team. When the first client, Jon Sommers, arrives, Susan begins the screening process:

Exercise 3-12: *Fill-in*
List the essential screening questions that Susan should ask.

_____

_____

_____

_____

Exercise 3-13: *Multiple-choice question*
When Susan asks Jon if he has had Guillain-Barré syndrome (GBS), he is confused and asks her, "I don't think so. What's that?" The best response that Susan can give is:
  A. Guillain-Barré syndrome is a rare metabolic disorder causing muscle weakness and sometimes paralysis.
  B. Guillain-Barré syndrome is a rare inflammatory vascular disorder of the peripheral veins and is characterized by numbness, tingling, weakness, or paralysis.
  C. Guillain-Barré syndrome is a neurological disorder in which a person's immune system attacks the peripheral nervous system, resulting in weakness and paralysis.
  D. Guillain-Barré syndrome is a respiratory condition. It is a form of bronchial inflammation resulting in increasing shortness of breath. The cause is unknown, but the trigger seems to be acute viral or bacterial infections.

Answers to this chapter begin on page 69.

Jon thinks about this for a minute and then asks, "You mean that if I had Guillain-Barré syndrome, I would not be able to get the flu shot?"

Exercise 3-14: *Multiple-choice question*
The best response to Jon's question is:
  A. If it has been 5 or more years since you had Guillain-Barré syndrome, you can get the flu shot.
  B. If you had Guillain-Barré syndrome within 6 weeks after a previous dose of influenza vaccine, it is very likely you cannot get a flu shot. It is best you speak to your doctor.
  C. Yes, that is correct. If you have had Guillain-Barré syndrome, you can never get the flu shot.
  D. Depending upon the severity of the Guillain-Barré syndrome you experienced, you may be able to get the flu shot but you should talk to your doctor.

Exercise 3-15: *Multiple-choice question*
A 72-year-old woman asks Ted, "What kinds of flu shots are available and recommended for me?"
The correct response would be:
  A. The regular flu shot is recommended for persons your age.
  B. The high-dose flu shot is recommended for persons your age.
  C. The intradermal flu shot is recommended for persons your age.
  D. The flu shot is not recommended for persons your age.

A family of five approaches the immunization station; the mother asks Susan about the vaccine and wants to know who in her family should get it. Susan does an assessment of the family.

Exercise 3-16: *Multiple-choice question*
Of the following members of this family, is there anyone who should not get the flu shot?
  A. The 36-year-old mother
  B. The 45-year-old father
  C. The 10-year-old boy
  D. The 5-month-old twins

The mother expresses concern regarding her twins' health. She tells Susan that she read somewhere that babies are particularly vulnerable and at high risk for complications related to the flu.

Answers to this chapter begin on page 69.

Exercise 3-17: *Multiple-choice question*

The best response for Susan to give to the mother is:

      A. We can administer the nasal vaccine to provide protection from the flu.

      B. Your babies are still protected by the natural immunity you transmitted during pregnancy.

      C. Your babies will be best protected if those around them receive the flu vaccine.

      D. The flu virus is not a danger to your babies.

 eResource 3-8: To learn more about protecting their babies from the flu, the couple listens to the CDC podcast: *Don't Get, Don't Spread: Seasonal Flu* by Dr. Joe Bresee: http://goo.gl/OuCe2

Theresa Snow is standing next to her friend Sally, who is getting a flu shot, turns to Ted and says, "I never get the flu shot. I have always been healthy and even when people around me get sick, I never do. I must be immune to the virus, I guess." Ted explains that flu virus changes year to year, and that is the reason that a new shot is provided each year. He continues a friendly conversation with the two women.

Exercise 3-18: *Multiple-choice question*

After further conversation with Theresa, he learns that she is the primary caregiver for two elderly relatives who have some chronic health problems. The correct response for Ted to give to the woman is:

      A. "People who are in frequent contact with individuals with chronic health problems are at higher risk for contracting the flu so these individuals should get the flu shot."

      B. "People with certain medical conditions including asthma, diabetes, and chronic lung disease are at higher risk for complications of influenza so their caregivers should get the flu shot."

      C. "Caregivers are at increased risk for contracting infections due to frequent and close contact with the infirm."

      D. "Elderly individuals living in the community are at greater risk of complications associated with the flu than their counterparts living in assisted living facilities."

 eResource 3-9: To provide supplemental instruction and reinforce the information he is providing Theresa, Ted pulls out his smartphone, opens a browser, and taps in the CDC web address to CDC Mobile: [Pathway: http://m.cdc.gov → "Diseases and Conditions" → "Seasonal Flu"]

Exercise 3-19: *Fill-in*

Who is at high risk for complications related to flu? (Please list)

_____

_____

_____

eResource 3-10: To find more information about people at high risk of developing flu-related complications, go to the CDC website: [Pathway: http://www.cdc.gov/flu → select "People at High Risk"]

Mr. Theodore Thompson, aged 70, approaches the nursing station. He wants to get the flu shot but has questions about the pneumonia shot. "I have heard that I should get this. What can you tell me about this? Am I at risk of getting pneumonia?" he asks Ted and Susan.

Exercise 3-20: *Multiple-choice question*
What would be the best response to give Mr. Thompson?
- A. "The greatest risk for an outbreak of pneumococcal pneumonia is among teenagers who have not yet received their booster shots."
- B. "The greatest risk for an outbreak of pneumococcal pneumonia is among people over age 65 who live in nursing homes and other extended care facilities."
- C. "The greatest risk for an outbreak of pneumococcal pneumonia is among children in early elementary school who have not been immunized."
- D. "The greatest risk for an outbreak of pneumococcal pneumonia is among adults aged 18 to 40 who have never been exposed to the agent before."

Mr. Thompson tells Susan that he lives alone but does go to the local senior center every day for lunch and to play cards with his friends.

Exercise 3-21: *Fill-in*
What is the recommendation for Mr. Thompson? Should he get the pneumonia vaccination?

_____

_____

 eResource 3-11: Ted provides Mr. Thompson with an adult immunization schedule: http://goo.gl/Pm4cd

Exercise 3-22: *Select all that apply*
Upon reviewing the document, Mr. Thompson sees that it is recommended that he also have the following immunization(s) because he is over the age of 60:
- ❑ HPV
- ❑ Zoster (shingles)
- ❑ MMR
- ❑ Hepatitis A
- ❑ Hepatitis B

Answers to this chapter begin on page 69.

Mr. Thompson asks Susan, "Some of the vaccines listed on this sheet are the vaccines that my grandchildren got before starting school. I was immunized as a child so why are these needed for adults?"

Exercise 3-23: *Multiple-choice question*

The best response for Susan to give is:

      A. "These immunizations are not needed for adults as they have naturally acquired immunity."

      B. "Immunity can begin to fade over time as we age."

      C. "Immunity, once acquired, lasts a lifetime."

      D. "The immunizations you received as a child should be sufficient to protect you from disease."

The station is equipped with a computer that has the CDC's Adult Scheduler tool downloaded and installed and a web-based interactive quiz. Ted uses the program to provide additional health education for Mr. Thompson.

    eResource 3-12:
    ■ Adult Immunization Scheduler: http://goo.gl/QrjLt
    ■ Adult and Adolescent Immunization Quiz: http://goo.gl/ImdXz

Susan and Ted are enjoying participating in the flu clinic and are excited about not only getting a lot of practice giving shots but also about having the opportunity to do patient teaching. It seems that people attending the fair are taking this opportunity to ask a wide variety of questions. For example, a 49-year-old man asked Ted about the swine flu. "Is this something I need to worry about this year? What can I do to protect myself against getting the swine flu?" Ted tells the man that since he is not at high risk for complications related to the regular flu, he is not "at risk"; however, if he does go to a fair where there are swine, there are things he can do to protect himself from getting sick.

Exercise 3-24: *Multiple-choice question*

Which of the following instructions are appropriate for Ted to give to the man?

      A. "You don't need to worry about the swine flu. The swine flu is a problem in underdeveloped countries only."

      B. "To maximize your protection against the swine flu, you should get the regular flu shot."

      C. "To maximize your protection against the swine flu, you should stay away from farms and minimize contact with pigs."

      D. "Get the flu vaccine. That will protect you from the swine flu."

At the next class meeting, the students discuss their experience of participating in the flu immunization program and how exciting it was to practice giving shots but also to interact with clients and to do health teaching.

Answers to this chapter begin on page 69.

Unfolding Case Study #2 ▬ Tuan Hoang—A Case of Tuberculosis

Tuan Hoang is a 39-year-old, recent immigrant from Vietnam and has been living and working in Houston, Texas, for the past 6 months. He works in his cousin's grocery store unloading delivery trucks and stocking the shelves. He comes to the free clinic at the health department complaining of a fever and a productive cough. He also reported that he has experienced weight loss, lack of energy, poor appetite, and night sweats. He thinks he has the flu and is asking for treatment. Sandra Parker, the nurse practitioner at the clinic, conducts a physical assessment and decides to test for tuberculosis (TB) because Tuan is presenting himself with typical symptoms associated with TB.

Exercise 3-25: *Multiple-choice question*
Symptoms of active TB pulmonary disease are:

    A. Cough, fever, night sweats, chest pain

    B. Lung cancer

    C. Orthostatic hypertension, cardiomegaly

    D. Weight loss, dependent edema, coughing

Warren is a nursing student shadowing Sandra for the day. Sandra discusses her assessment with Warren to help him understand why she has decided to test Tuan for TB.

Exercise 3-26: *Select all that apply*
Testing Tuan for TB is warranted because:

    ❑ He is from a country that has a high incidence of TB

    ❑ He has a fever and productive cough

    ❑ He is a recent immigrant

    ❑ He has experienced weight loss, lack of energy, poor appetite, and night sweats

Warren remembers that he was required to take a two-step process. Sandra orders a chest x-ray and obtains a sputum sample. She tells Warren that the presence of acid-fast-bacilli (AFB) on a sputum smear often indicates TB disease.
    Sandra asks Warren, "What tests can confirm the diagnosis of TB?"

Exercise 3-27: *Select all that apply*
When screening for TB, there are several tests commonly utilized. However, a definitive diagnosis of TB can only be confirmed by:

    ❑ TB blood test

    ❑ Mantoux tuberculin skin test (TST)

Answers to this chapter begin on page 69.

❑ Chest x-ray

❑ AFB sputum smear

❑ Sputum culture

❑ A thorough medical history

Sandra and Warren continue to discuss the case. She tells Warren that the Mantoux test (TST) is used frequently in the clinic to screen for TB—particularly among individuals who are not presenting symptoms—however, it is important to conduct a comprehensive medical history prior to ordering any tests, particularly for TB. Warren is surprised by this. He asks her "Why is that important?"

Exercise 3-28: *Select all that apply*

Sandra explains that there are several factors in which a TST is contraindicated, and therefore it is important to ask the client specifically regarding any history of the following:

❑ A recent viral illness such as measles, mumps, rubella, or influenza

❑ Recent travel outside of the United States

❑ Any recent immunizations such as yellow fever, varicella, and/or the MMR vaccine in the last 6 weeks

❑ A positive TB test in the past

❑ Steroid use

❑ Elevated temperature

❑ A suppressed immune system

Sandra asks Warren, "What does a positive TST mean? Does it mean that the patient has TB?"

Exercise 3-29: *Multiple-choice question*

Warren thinks for a minute before responding. A positive TST means that a person has:

A. The TB disease

B. Been exposed to TB germs

C. Has an allergy to the vaccine

D. Is from another country

Exercise 3-30: *True or false*

Sandra asks a follow-up question. Does a positive TST mean that a person is contagious?

A. True, a positive TST means that the person is contagious.

B. False, a positive TST does not mean that the person is contagious.

Answers to this chapter begin on page 69.

Sandra also uses this opportunity to help Warren understand the public health concerns regarding TB in the community. She explains that even though the incidence of TB in the United States has declined, it is still a public health concern, and there is a public health initiative under way to reduce the incidence of TB in the country—with the goal of total elimination. Warren remembers that this was discussed in class. A classmate had asked the instructor, "What makes it so hard to eliminate TB?"

Exercise 3-31: *Multiple-choice question*

The instructor had explained that the CDC (2005) has identified several factors that are interfering with the efforts to eliminate TB. These include all of the following except:

    A. Prevalence of TB among foreign-born persons residing in the United States

    B. Lack of effective treatment regimens

    C. Delays in detecting and reporting cases of pulmonary TB

    D. Deficiencies in protecting contacts of persons with infectious TB and in preventing and responding to TB outbreaks

    E. Persistence of a substantial population of persons living in the United States with latent TB infection who are at risk for progression to TB disease

    F. Maintaining clinical and public health expertise in an era of declining TB incidence

The results of the chest x-ray and rapid test are back and indicate that Tuan very likely has TB.

Exercise 3-32: *Multiple-choice question*

Sandra asks Warren, "So, Tuan has the signs and symptoms of TB disease and both the chest x-ray and rapid test indicate likelihood of TB. A sputum sample has been sent to the lab for culture, but will not be back for 24 hours. What is our next step?"

    A. Wait until the culture results confirming the diagnosis of TB are back

    B. Begin Tuan on TB disease treatment

    C. Consult with the public health department

    D. Test him next year

Sandra tells Tuan that he will be started on medication to treat TB. She explains that his symptoms, the chest x-ray, and sputum smear indicate that he has TB but that it will not be officially confirmed until the culture results come back tomorrow. Tuan has a lot of questions that Warren and Sandra answer. His first question is, "What is TB actually and what causes it?" Sandra tells Tuan, "TB is a serious disease caused by the germ *Mycobacterium tuberculosis*. TB can hurt your lungs. The good news is that TB can be prevented and it can be cured."

She tells Tuan that because he is coughing and has other symptoms of active TB, he is contagious and will need to be in isolation, not visit family or friends, and stay out of public places. She tells him that she has to ask a few questions to make sure this is safe. Tuan is confused, "Don't you have to go to the hospital if you have TB?" Sandra replies, "In the past, patients used to, but now, if certain criteria are met, the patient can be at home instead of in the hospital."

Exercise 3-33: *Select all that apply*
Which of the following criteria must be met for a patient with suspected/confirmed TB to be on home isolation?

❑ Patient can speak and read English.

❑ Patient has a stable residence at verified address.

❑ Patient can care for himself or herself and not require hospitalization for other medical conditions.

❑ Patient does not live with immunocompromised persons.

❑ Patient has someone at home who can take care of him or her.

❑ Patient does not live with TST-negative children.

❑ Environmental assessment finds the home compatible with effective isolation.

❑ Patient does not live in a congregate setting such as shelter, nursing home, or single-room-occupancy hotel.

Sandra tells Tuan that he must agree to comply with risk-reduction behaviors until the doctor says he is no longer contagious and that he will need to go to the outpatient TB Program Clinic daily to receive his medication as part of a Direct Observation Therapy (DOT) program. She explains that he must wear a mask when he is out in public during the time when he is still contagious (CDC, Division of Tuberculosis Elimination, 2011b).

Exercise 3-34: *Fill-in*
What are some of the other criteria for including Tuan in this program?

_____

_____

_____

Exercise 3-35: *Multiple-choice question*
Tuan asks "How did I get TB?" Warren tells Tuan that the *Mycobacterium tuberculosis* is usually transmitted by:

A. Semen and other body fluids

B. Food and water

C. Used needles

D. Airborne droplets

Sandra further explains to Tuan that it is likely that he was in close proximity to someone who had active TB and was contagious. Now, because he is coughing productively, he is also contagious. Therefore, to protect others, he will need

Answers to this chapter begin on page 69.

to be started on medication right away. She tells him that he will need to be on medications for a long time (CDC, Division of Tuberculosis Elimination, 2011c). She also tells him that she will make arrangements for a public health nurse to make a home visit to assess family members for illness. She asks Tuan to recall all the places he has gone to since he has begun feeling ill and started coughing. She tells him that the three main places that people are usually in close contact with others are home, work or school, and social settings. Tuan says, "I work long hours at the grocery store. I just work and go home." Sandra realizes that it is very likely that the public health nurse will only need to focus on Tuan's home and workplace. She asks Tuan for a list of his close contacts at work because they too need to be tested for TB. Tuan is worried that if the people he works with find out he has TB, he will be fired. Sandra assures Tuan that his privacy will be protected and that his preferences can be accommodated (*Morbidity and Mortality Weekly Report [MMWR]*, 2005; NYC Department of Health and Mental Hygiene, Bureau of TB Control, n.d.).

 eResource 3-13: Sandra gives Tuan a pamphlet that explains the process in more detail: http://goo.gl/9KAxX

Tuan asks Sandra, "So, what's next? How is this TB treated?" Sandra begins to explain the treatment regimen.

Exercise 3-36: *True or false*
The standard treatment for active TB infection is a combination therapy of four drugs: isoniazid (INH), rifampin (RIF), ethambutol (EMB), and pyrazinamide (PZA) taken daily for 9 months.
    A. True
    B. False

Sandra also tells Tuan that when he goes home, he will need to participate in a directly observed therapy (DOT) program. She explains that it is very important that the medication is taken as directed because the bacteria have the opportunity to develop resistance to the drugs and become much more difficult to treat. Therefore, most treatment programs require that a health care professional watch clients take every dose. She explains that it is the DOT program that helps a patient complete the program successfully and can be easily incorporated into Tuan's daily routine. The DOT worker can come to his home or—when he is no longer contagious—even to his workplace or a park, wherever it is convenient.

Exercise 3-37: *True or false*
Directly observed therapy (DOT) involves viewing taking medications to ensure compliance. This is an example of tertiary prevention.
    A. True
    B. False

Sandra explains to Tuan that the public health nurse working with the TB Control Program will be assessing Tuan's family and coworkers for TB. She explains that there are two forms of TB: TB disease and latent TB infection (LTBI). She tells Tuan that because he has symptoms of illness, he has TB disease. He is confused and asks more questions about latent TB (CDC, Division of Tuberculosis Elimination, 2012a).

Exercise 3-38: *Multiple-choice question*

The difference between latent TB infection and TB disease is that:

    A. People with latent TB infection are not infectious, whereas people with TB disease are sometimes infectious.

    B. Only TB disease can be detected by a tuberculin skin test; latent TB infection cannot.

    C. People with latent TB infection are infectious, whereas people with TB disease are not.

    D. Latent TB infection is curable but TB disease is not.

Exercise 3-39: *Fill-in*

Indicate which of the following are characteristics of latent TB infection (LTBI) or TB disease or both (B)?

    _____ Tubercle bacilli are inactive in the body.

    _____ Individuals are often infectious before treatment.

    _____ Usually the chest x-ray is normal.

    _____ Sputum smears and cultures are negative.

    _____ Individuals do not have symptoms.

    _____ Individuals are not infectious.

    _____ Tubercle bacilli are active in the body.

    _____ The TST and QFT-G results are usually positive.

    _____ Usually the chest x-ray is abnormal.

    _____ Sputum smears and cultures are usually positive for *M. tuberculosis*.

    _____ Individuals have symptoms.

Sandra continues to provide patient teaching to Tuan, telling him about the standard treatment for TB infection and what he can expect. She gives Tuan the risk reduction guidelines and reviews these with him:

1. Do NOT receive visitors at home or visit the homes of others.

2. Do NOT care for children, work outside the home, or take a trip without the doctor's permission.

3. Avoid public transportation.

4. Cover the mouth and nose when coughing or sneezing.

5. Prevent coughs by drinking warm fluids and by sucking on soothing candies.

6. Limit the time spent in common household areas (such as the bathroom or kitchen) and spend as much time alone.

7. Open a window and use a fan to blow air outside if possible.

8. Wear a surgical mask when spending time in a space that is also used by others (Nilsen, n.d., p. 19).

Answers to this chapter begin on page 69.

Sandra completes her documentation and sends the required reports to the City Health Department's TB Control Program.

Maria Torres works as a public health nurse working in the city's TB Control Program. She is assigned to do a home assessment. She knows that Tuan lives with his cousin in a small two-bedroom apartment. While being interviewed, Tuan tells Maria that he doesn't really like to take medications and usually takes herbal remedies. He asks her if he can take an alternative herbal regimen to treat his TB.

Exercise 3-40: *Multiple-choice question*
The appropriate response for Maria to make is:
A. Tell Tuan that he can continue with his alternative herbal regimen along with the TB medication.
B. Tell Tuan that there is a possibility that he can take his alternative herbal regimen as long as he continues his TB drugs, but these need to be reviewed by the doctor first.
C. Tell Tuan he cannot take an alternative herbal regimen and take only his TB pills.
D. Tell Tuan to adhere to the regimen that makes him feel best.

Seizing the window of opportunity presented by Tuan's questions, Maria begins patient teaching regarding the medication regimen.

 eResource 3-14: She provides Tuan with a pamphlet, *Staying on Track with TB Medicine:* http://goo.gl/So5LF

Maria tells Tuan, "You have TB disease. It will be very important for you to take your medication as directed by your doctor." She goes on to explain that "If you have TB disease, you must remember that TB germs die very slowly. Even if you feel better after a few weeks on the TB medicines, it does not mean all the TB germs are dead. Treating TB takes months. Staying on your medicine the way you are supposed to is the only way to cure TB" (CDC Division of Tuberculosis Elimination, 2011a, p. 4).

Maria also needs to interview and assess Tuan's contacts. She knows that prior to doing the contact investigation and interviews, she needs to determine the infectious period. The CDC states that this is "a time frame during which potential exposure to others may have occurred while the patient was infectious or able to transmit TB. Often, the beginning of the infectious period is when the onset of symptoms occurs, especially coughing. Local or state standards should be used to determine the beginning of the infectious period. Some health department guidelines denote a specified period prior to the patient recollection of the onset of symptoms, particularly coughing" (CDC Division of Tuberculosis Elimination, 2006, p. 4).

Exercise 3-41: *Multiple-choice question*
Maria remembers that for the purpose of the contact investigation, the end of the infectious period is determined by all of the following except:
A. Frequency and intensity of cough have improved
B. Patient feels better

Answers to this chapter begin on page 69.

C. Patient has been receiving adequate treatment for at least 2 weeks

D. Reduction of the grade of the AFB sputum smear or negative sputum smears

E. A and C

F. A, B, and C

G. A, C, and D

Maria first interviews Tuan at his apartment to determine individuals who may have come in contact with him during the period he was infectious.

Exercise 3-42: *Multiple-choice question*

When trying to determine individuals who may have come in contact with Tuan during the infectious period, how far back should Maria ask the index patient to recall?

A. 6 months

B. 3 months

C. The designated time of the infectious period based on local or state standards

D. When medications were initiated

Tuan reports that the only people he has been in direct contact with during this period were his family and coworkers in his cousin's grocery store.

Before Maria goes to visit Tuan's contacts, she remembers the training she had previously regarding conducting interviews.

 eResource 3-15: Before Maria makes her home visit to do a home assessment, she reviews
- The CDC guidelines: http://goo.gl/Pfi1j
- The *Effective TB Interviewing for Contact Investigation: Self-Study Modules:* http://goo.gl/HFD8K

Maria is also prepared to interview and assess Tuan's family and coworkers. She knows that she will need to administer the Mantoux tuberculin skin test to Tuan's family and coworkers to assess for latent TB.

 eResource 3-16: To learn more about this procedure, listen to/watch the CDC Pod/Vodcast:
- Audio only: http://goo.gl/UiMFP
- Video: http://goo.gl/EVTtR

Maria realizes that depending upon the results of the test, it is very likely that someone may need to receive treatment for latent TB infection.

Exercise 3-43: *Fill-in*

What is latent TB infection and how is it definitively diagnosed?

_____

_____

Exercise 3-44: *Multiple-choice question*

The standard treatment for latent TB infection is to:

A. Give isoniazid daily for 9 months.

B. Give rifampin and isoniazid daily for 18 months.

C. Closely monitor the patient's health status and then give isoniazid only if TB disease develops.

D. Treat with a regimen of four drugs for 6 months.

E. Treat with a regimen of three drugs for 12 months.

 eResource 3-17: To learn more about specific treatment protocols for latent TB infection, go to: http://goo.gl/N7HDK

When Maria visits Tuan's home, she meets with Tuan's sister Kim-Ly Mai who lives next door with her family. Kim-Ly, 42, has lots of questions about TB and how this disease affects people. Maria reviews the basics of transmission and pathogenicity of TB. Kim-Ly understands that TB is transmitted via droplets, but has other questions regarding the effect of TB on the body.

 eResource 3-18: To provide more information about latent TB and how to prevent TB disease from developing, Maria shows Kim-Ly a video: *You Can Beat TB,* http://youtu.be/wlT_UvKQlD4

Exercise 3-45: *Multiple-choice question*

Which of the following statements about TB is true?

A. TB is caused by a virus.

B. TB only affects the lungs.

C. TB can be fatal.

D. TB is highly contagious.

E. Everyone infected with TB gets sick.

Kim-Ly is concerned that others in the household will be at risk for getting TB. She is very concerned about her 5-month-old grandson, Huu. Maria asks about other members in the household to identify who is at risk, but explains that since Tuan has been diagnosed with TB disease, it is important that all members of the household be tested for TB. She explains that some people are more at risk because they have health conditions that make their body weaker and less resistant to the bacteria.

Exercise 3-46: *Select all that apply*

Kim-Ly tells Maria the names and ages of the other people currently living in the home. Which members are particularly at risk for developing TB disease?

❑ Soo-Ye, Tuan and Kim-Ly's grandmother (83 years)

❑ Chinh-Dahn, Tuan and Kim-Ly's father (66 years)

❑ Trang, Kim-Ly's husband (48 years)

Answers to this chapter begin on page 69.

❑ Linh, Kim-Ly's daughter (22 years)

❑ Trong Tri, Linh's husband (23 years)

❑ Thomas, Kim-Ly's son (20 years)

❑ Huu, Linh's son (5 months)

Kim-Ly tells Maria that while she is worried about her family catching TB from Tuan, "None of them are sick so maybe I am worrying for nothing." Maria tells Kim-Ly that it is possible to have TB but not be sick. She explains that latent TB infection (LTBI) is when TB is in the body but the body is strong enough—for the time being—to fight off the disease. Sometimes LTBI can be present for years and not cause a problem. Maria also tells Kim-Ly that there are some conditions that appear to increase the risk of developing TB disease.

Exercise 3-47: *Multiple-choice question*
Which of the following conditions increase the risk of developing TB disease?

    A. Cardiac disease

    B. Kidney transplant

    C. COPD

    D. Asthma

 eResource 3-19: To learn more about current treatment of latent TB, Kim-Ly listens to the CDC podcast: http://goo.gl/41wZ8

Kim-Ly tells Maria she feels better now. She is still worried about the test results, but now that she understands how TB can be managed and cured, she knows she can handle it. Maria makes an appointment to follow up with Kim-Ly at the clinic in a few days.

Unfolding Case Study #3   Thomas

Maria realizes that Tuan's diagnosis of TB disease has placed his family at risk because they live in very close quarters in a very small three-bedroom bungalow. She plans to interview each of the adults in the household privately. Thomas is Tuan's nephew and lives in the same home with Tuan and their extended family. Maria asks Thomas about his health and how he has been feeling. She asks if he has any medical conditions that might place him at risk.

 eResource 3-20: Prior to making the home visit, Maria consults the Agency for Healthcare Research and Quality (AHRQ) National Guidelines Clearing house for the latest practice guidelines: [Pathway: http://guideline.gov → enter "latent tb" into the search field → scroll down to access and review the most current guidelines]

Answers to this chapter begin on page 69.

Exercise 3-48: *Multiple-choice question*
Which of the following health conditions places a person at the highest risk of developing TB disease after becoming infected?

     A. Fatigue

     B. Less than ideal body weight

     C. Pneumonia

     D. HIV infection

     E. Diabetes

Maria also asks Thomas about his lifestyle practices. She knows that people who have conditions that make the body weaker have a reduced ability to fight the TB germ. She explains to him that it is important that she asks these questions because conditions that weaken the immune system, such as HIV and AIDS, would increase the risk of contracting TB disease. Thomas tells Maria that he is gay but is not in a relationship currently (CDC, Division of Tuberculosis Elimination, 2012b).

Exercise 3-49: *Multiple-choice question*
HIV is a retrovirus that

     A. Attacks the immune system destroying T-cells or CD-4 cells necessary for fighting infection

     B. Attacks the immune system destroying beta cells necessary for fighting infection

     C. Attacks the immune system, incapacitating all cells that are necessary for fighting infection

     D. None of the above

 eResource 3-21: Maria provides Thomas with additional information to help him understand the importance of getting treatment by showing him a brief video in which Dr. Kenneth Castro, Director of the Division of Tuberculosis Elimination, explains why it is important for people living with HIV to be tested for TB and treated: http://goo.gl/pGI5p

After listening to the video clip, Thomas asks the nurse, "So, what can I do to protect myself and my family?" Maria responds, "It is important to remember that when you have HIV infection, your system is weak, so you catch things pretty easily. It is hard enough dealing with HIV so we want to make sure that you don't get TB."

 eResource 3-22: Maria also provides additional information regarding TB testing, treating TB infection, and treating TB disease when a person has HIV infection:

     ■ Tuberculosis: The Connection between TB and HIV (the AIDS virus): http://goo.gl/Tvwnp

     ■ Take Steps to Control TB Tuberculosis When You Have HIV: http://goo.gl/UHZ8V

Answers to this chapter begin on page 69.

Maria makes an appointment with Thomas for a follow-up visit in the clinic to read the test. As she leaves the home, she thinks about the visit and wonders if Tuan will follow through with his treatment regimen. She knows that it is a challenge to balance individual autonomy against community protection. She hopes that Tuan will follow through with his promise.

Answers to this chapter begin on page 69.

Answers

Exercise 3-1: *Fill-in*

1. What factors contributed to the spread of the flu in 1918?

   a. **The lack of a flu vaccine**

   b. **Failure to close public places and public meetings during the pandemic**

   c. **Misconceptions about the transmission of the flu**

2. What factors or conditions put a person at risk for contracting the flu?

   a. **Chronic diseases such as diabetes**

3. What is the most effective way to protect against the flu?

   a. **Get the flu and pneumonia shots**

Exercise 3-2: *True or false*

A person who gets the flu shot is immediately protected against the flu.

A. True

B. False

Exhibit 3-1: Answer Details

The protection against the flu builds over a 2-week period.

Exercise 3-3: *Select all that apply*

In regard to routine immunizations, which of the following is not an appropriate procedure for the health care provider to follow?

☒ **Always administer vaccines as indicated on the immunization schedule.**

❑ Avoid missing opportunities to vaccinate.

☒ **Avoid administering immunizations to pregnant women.**

❑ Screen patients each time prior to vaccinating.

Exhibit 3-2: Answer Details

Administration of vaccines may be deferred due to high fevers.

Exercise 3-4: *Select all that apply*

Which of the following criteria is a contraindication for administering the diphtheria, tetanus, pertussis (DTaP) vaccine?

❑ Temperature of 104°F following previous administration of the DTP or DTaP vaccine

❑ Family history of seizures

☒ **Encephalopathy of unknown etiology within 7 days following previous administration of the DTP or DTaP vaccine**

❑ Family history of sudden infant death syndrome

❑ Family history of an adverse event after DTP or DTaP administration

❑ Immunodeficient family member or household contact

Exercise 3-5: *Multiple-choice question*
Other factors affecting the severity of the flu season include all of the following except:
A. How much flu vaccine is available—NO, this is a reason for increased cases.
B. Route along which the vaccine is administered—YES, this does not have an effect.
C. When the flu vaccine is available—NO, this is a factor.
D. How many people get vaccinated—NO, this is the most significant variable.

Exercise 3-6: *Multiple-choice question*
Which of the following activities/strategies can be utilized to prevent or minimize widespread influenza infection?
A. Conduct community outreach program—NO, this is a factor, but not the only one.
B. Offer flu shot clinics—NO, this is a factor, but not the only one.
C. Teach regarding proper hand washing—NO, this is a factor, but not the only one.
D. Take antiviral medications as prescribed by physician—NO, this is a factor, but not the only one.
E. All of the above—YES, all of them
F. A, B and C—NO, these are factors, but not the only ones.

Exhibit 3-3: Answer Details

"Studies show that flu antiviral drugs work best for treatment when they are started within 2 days of getting sick, but starting them later can still be helpful, especially if the sick person has a high-risk health or is very sick from the flu."

Source: CDC (2012), p. 3.

Exercise 3-7: *Select all that apply*
Which of the following groups is (are) particularly vulnerable to flu-related complications?

☒ **Young children**

❑ Nursing babies

☒ **People over age 65**

❑ Adolescents

☒ **Pregnant women**

❑ Recent immigrants

☒ **People with asthma**

☒ **People with diabetes**

Exercise 3-8: *Multiple-choice question*
Which of the following are contraindications for administering the influenza "live" attenuated (LAIV) vaccine?

A. Pregnant or breastfeeding family member or household contact

B. Breastfeeding

C. Children who are on aspirin therapy

D. Health care workers that care for patients in protective isolation

E. Contacts of persons with chronic medical conditions

Exercise 3-9: *Multiple-choice question*
Which of the following definitions from the CDC (2007) accurately describes passive immunity?

A. "Resistance developed in response to an antigen (i.e., an infecting agent or vaccine), usually characterized by the presence of an antibody produced by the host"—NO, it is not produced by the host.

B. "The resistance to an infectious agent of an entire group or community as a result of a substantial proportion of the population being immune to the agent"—NO, the immunity is lacking.

C. "Immunity conferred by an antibody produced in another host"—YES

Exercise 3-10: *Multiple-choice question*
Which would be considered a host in the chain of infection?

A. Human—NO, it is *Escherichia coli*.

B. Excessive heat—NO, it is *Escherichia coli*.

C. Overcrowding—NO, it is *Escherichia coli*.

D. *Escherichia coli*—YES

Exercise 3-11: *Multiple-choice question*
An individual acquires artificial immunity by:

A. Being vaccinated (rather than via exposure)—YES

B. Previous infection with the disease—NO, this doesn't acquire artificial immunity.

C. Previous exposure to the disease—NO, this doesn't acquire artificial immunity.

D. From the body's antigen-antibody response to infection—NO, this doesn't acquire artificial immunity.

E. Having a compromised immune system—NO, this doesn't acquire artificial immunity.

Exercise 3-12: *Fill-in*

List the essential screening questions that Susan should ask.

1. <u>**Is the person to be vaccinated sick today?**</u>

2. <u>**Does the person to be vaccinated have an allergy to eggs or to a component**</u>
   <u>**of the vaccine?**</u>

3. <u>**Has the person to be vaccinated ever had a serious reaction to influenza vac-**</u>
   <u>**cine in the past?**</u>

4. <u>**Has the person to be vaccinated ever had Guillain-Barré syndrome?**</u>
   <u>**(Immunization Action Coalition, 2012, p. 1)**</u>

Exercise 3-13: *Multiple-choice question*

When Susan asks Jon if he has had Guillain-Barré syndrome (GBS), he is confused and asks her, "I don't think so. What's that?" The best response that Susan can give is:

A. "Guillain-Barré syndrome is a rare metabolic disorder causing muscle weakness and sometimes paralysis."—NO, it is a neurological disease.

B. "Guillain-Barré syndrome is a rare inflammatory vascular disorder of the peripheral veins and is characterized by numbness, tingling, weakness, or paralysis."—NO, it is a neurological disease.

C. "Guillain-Barré syndrome is a neurological disorder in which a person's immune system attacks the peripheral nervous system, resulting in weakness and paralysis."—YES

D. "Guillain-Barré syndrome is a respiratory condition. It is a form of bronchial inflammation resulting in increasing shortness of breath. The cause is unknown, but the trigger seems to be acute viral or bacterial infections."—NO, it is a neurological disease.

Exercise 3-14:

The best response to Jon's question is:

A. "If it has been 5 or more years since you had Guillain-Barré syndrome, you can get the flu shot."—NO, this is not sound advice.

B. "If you had Guillain-Barré syndrome within 6 weeks after a previous dose of influenza vaccine, it is very likely you cannot get a flu shot. It is best you speak to your doctor."—YES, this is correct.

C. "Yes, that is correct. If you have had Guillain-Barré syndrome, you can never get the flu shot."—NO, this is not true.

D. "Depending upon the severity of the Guillain-Barré syndrome you experienced, you may be able to get the flu shot, but you should talk to your doctor."—NO, this is not correct either.

Exercise 3-15: *Multiple-choice question*

A 72-year-old woman asks Ted, "What kinds of flu shots are available and recommended for me?"

The correct response would be:

A. "The regular flu shot is recommended for persons your age."—NO, this is not correct.

B. "The high-dose flu shot is recommended for persons your age."—YES

C. "The intradermal flu shot is recommended for persons your age."—NO, this is not true.

D. "The flu shot is not recommended for persons your age."—NO, it is not the regular dose that is recommended.

Exercise 3-16: *Multiple-choice question*

Of the following members of this family, is there anyone who should not get the flu shot?

A. The 36-year-old mother—NO, this person should receive the flu shot.

B. The 45-year-old father—NO, this person should receive the flu shot.

C. The 10-year-old boy—NO, this person should receive the flu shot.

D. The 5-month-old twins—YES, too young

Exercise 3-17: *Multiple-choice question*

The best response for Susan to give to the mother is:

A. "We can administer the nasal vaccine to provide protection from the flu."—NO, this is not the appropriate route of administration for this situation.

B. "Your babies are still protected by the natural immunity you transmitted during pregnancy."—NO, this is not true, they are not protected.

C. "Your babies will be best protected if those around them receive the flu vaccine."—YES, this is the best response.

D. "The flu virus is not a danger to your babies."—NO, it is a danger.

Exercise 3-18: *Multiple-choice question*

After further conversation with Theresa, he learns that she is the primary caregiver for two elderly relatives who have some chronic health problems. The correct response for Ted to give to the woman is:

A. "People who are in frequent contact with individuals with chronic health problems are at higher risk for contracting the flu, so these individuals should get the flu shot."—NO, the person with the chronic illness is more at risk.

B. "People with certain medical conditions including asthma, diabetes, and chronic lung disease are at higher risk for complications of influenza, so their caregivers should get the flu shot."—YES

C. "Caregivers are at increased risk for contracting infections due to frequent and close contact with the infirm."—NO, the person with the chronic illness is more at risk.

D. "Elderly individuals living in the community are at greater risk of complications associated with the flu than their counterparts living in assisted living facilities."—NO, the person with the chronic illness is more at risk, not just because of the fact that they live in the community.

Exercise 3-19: *Fill-in*

Who is at high risk for complications related to the flu? (Please list)

People at high risk for developing flu-related complications:

- **Children younger than 5, but especially children younger than 2 years old**
- **Adults 65 years of age and older**
- **Pregnant women**
- **Also, American Indians and Alaskan Natives seem to be at higher risk of flu complications**

People who have medical conditions including:

- **Asthma**
- **Neurological and neurodevelopmental conditions (including disorders of the brain, spinal cord, peripheral nerve, and muscle such as cerebral palsy, epilepsy [seizure disorders], stroke, intellectual disability [mental retardation], moderate to severe developmental delay, muscular dystrophy, or spinal cord injury)**
- **Chronic lung disease (such as chronic obstructive pulmonary disease [COPD] and cystic fibrosis)**
- **Heart disease (such as congenital heart disease, congestive heart failure, and coronary artery disease)**
- **Blood disorders (such as sickle cell disease)**
- **Endocrine disorders (such as diabetes mellitus)**
- **Kidney disorders**
- **Liver disorders**
- **Metabolic disorders (such as inherited metabolic disorders and mitochondrial disorders)**
- **Weakened immune system due to disease or medication (such as people with HIV, or AIDS, or cancer, or those on chronic steroids)**
- **People younger than 19 years of age who are receiving long-term aspirin therapy**
- **People who are morbidly obese (body mass index, or BMI, of 40 or greater) (CDC, 2011, p. 1)**

Exercise 3-20: *Multiple-choice question*

What would be the best response to give Mr. Thompson?

A. "The greatest risk for an outbreak of pneumococcal pneumonia is among teenagers who have not yet received their booster shots."—NO, this is not true.

B. **"The greatest risk for an outbreak of pneumococcal pneumonia is among people over age 65 who live in nursing homes and other extended care facilities."—YES, this is the population at risk.**

C. "The greatest risk for an outbreak of pneumococcal pneumonia is among children in early elementary school who have not been immunized."—NO, this is not a greatest risk population.

D. "The greatest risk for an outbreak of pneumococcal pneumonia is among adults aged 18 to 40 who have never been exposed to the agent before."—NO, healthy adults are not in the risk group.

Exercise 3-21: *Fill-in*

What is the recommendation for Mr. Thompson? Should he get the pneumonia vaccination?

The elderly over age 65, particularly those who live in extended-care facilities or visit places/community settings where other older adults congregate—such as senior centers—should receive the pneumonia vaccination. One shot after age 65 will protect you for the rest of your life.

Exercise 3-22: *Select all that apply*

Upon reviewing the document, Mr. Thompson sees that it is recommended that he also have the following immunization(s) because he is over the age of 60:

❏ HPV

☒ **Zoster (shingles)**

❏ MMR

❏ Hepatitis A

❏ Hepatitis B

Exercise 3-23: *Multiple-choice question*

The best response for Susan to give is:

A. "These immunizations are not needed for adults as they have naturally acquired immunity."—NO, this is not true because immunity can decrease over time.

B. **"Immunity can begin to fade over time as we age."—YES**

C. "Immunity, once acquired, lasts a lifetime."—NO, this is not true.

D. "The immunizations you received as a child should be sufficient to protect you from disease."—NO, this is not true.

<h3 style="text-align:center">Exhibit 3-4: Answer Details</h3>

Vaccines received as children do not always protect individuals for the rest of their lives. This is because some adults missed being vaccinated when they were children, some of the newer vaccinations weren't available back then, immunity can begin to fade over time, and as we age we become more vulnerable to infection.

Exercise 3-24: *Multiple-choice question*

Which of the following instructions are appropriate for Ted to give to the man?

A. "You don't need to worry about the swine flu. The swine flu is a problem in under-developed countries only."—NO, this is not true.

B. "To maximize your protection against the swine flu, you should get the regular flu shot."—NO, the regular flu shot does not protect against swine flu.

C. "To maximize your protection against the swine flu, you should stay away from farms and minimize contact with pigs."—YES

D. "Get the flu vaccine. That will protect you from the swine flu."—NO, this is not true.

Exhibit 3-5: Answer Details

Additional precautions

- Don't take food or drink into pig areas; don't eat, drink, or put anything in your mouth in pig areas

- Get the flu vaccine

- Wash your hands often with soap and running water before and after exposure to pigs. If soap and water are not available, use an alcohol-based hand rub

- Avoid close contact with pigs that look or act ill

- Minimize contact with pigs and swine barns

Exercise 3-25: *Multiple-choice question*

Symptoms of active TB pulmonary disease are:

A. Cough, fever, night sweats, chest pain—YES, these are the classic manifestations.

B. Lung cancer—NO

C. Orthostatic hypertension, cardiomegaly—NO

D. Weight loss, dependent edema, coughing—NO

Exercise 3-26: *Select all that apply*

Testing Tuan for TB is warranted because:

☐ He is from a country that has a high incidence of TB—NO, the mere fact that he is from a country that has a high incidence does not warrant the TB test.

☒ **He has a fever and productive cough**

☒ **He is a recent immigrant**

☒ **He has experienced weight loss, lack of energy, poor appetite, and night sweats**

Exercise 3-27: *Select all that apply*

When screening for TB, there are several tests commonly utilized. However, a definitive diagnosis of TB can only be confirmed by:

❑ TB blood test

❑ Mantoux tuberculin skin test (TST)

❑ Chest x-ray

❑ AFB Sputum smear

☒ **Sputum culture**

❑ A thorough medical history

Exhibit 3-6: Answer Details

"The presence of acid-fast-bacilli (AFB) on a sputum smear or other specimen often indicates TB disease. Acid-fast microscopy is easy and quick, but it does not confirm a diagnosis of TB because some acid-fast-bacilli are not *M. tuberculosis*. Therefore, a culture is done on all initial samples to confirm the diagnosis."

Source: CDC Division of Tuberculosis Elimination (October 28, 2011b), p. 7.

Exercise 3-28: *Select all that apply*

Sandra explains that there are several factors in which a Mantoux test (TST) is contraindicated; therefore it is important to ask the client specifically regarding any history of the following:

☒ **A recent viral illness such as measles, mumps, rubella, or influenza**

❑ Recent travel outside the United States

☒ **Any recent immunizations such as yellow fever, varicella, and/or the MMR vaccine in the last 6 weeks**

☒ **A positive TB test in the past**

☒ **Steroid use**

❑ Elevated temperature

☒ **A suppressed immune system**

Exercise 3-29: *Multiple-choice question*

Warren thinks for a minute before responding. A positive TST means that a person has:

A. The TB disease—NO, this is just a screening test and does not confirm disease.

B. Been exposed to TB germs—YES

C. Has an allergy to the vaccine—NO, an allergic reaction to the TST would not present in a manner that would resemble an allergic response. A positive TST test confirms exposure to the *M. tuberculosis*.

D. Is from another country—NO, country of origin has no bearing on these results. While individuals from some countries may have a higher incidence of TB and may have a positive TST test, individuals from the US may also have a positive TST test.

Exercise 3-30: *True or false*

Sandra asks a follow-up question. Does a positive TST mean that a person is contagious?

A. True, a positive TST means that the person is contagious—NO

B. False, a positive TST does not mean that the person is contagious—YES

Exercise 3-31: *Multiple-choice question*

The instructor had explained that the CDC (2005) has identified several factors that are interfering with the efforts to eliminate TB. These include all of the following except:

A. Prevalence of TB among foreign-born persons residing in the United States—NO, this is a true consideration.

B. Lack of effective treatment regimens—YES, this is not the consideration in the United States.

C. Delays in detecting and reporting cases of pulmonary TB—NO, this is a true consideration.

D. Deficiencies in protecting contacts of persons with infectious TB and in preventing and responding to TB outbreaks—NO, this is a true consideration.

E. Persistence of a substantial population of persons living in the United States with LTBI who are at risk for progression to TB disease—NO, this is a true consideration.

F. Maintaining clinical and public health expertise in an era of declining TB incidence—NO, this is a true consideration.

Exercise 3-32: *Multiple-choice question*

Sandra asks Warren, "So, Tuan has the signs and symptoms of TB disease and both the chest x-ray and rapid test indicate the likelihood of TB. A sputum sample has been sent to the lab for culture but will not be back for 24 hours. What is our next step?"

A. Wait until the culture results confirming the diagnosis of TB are back—NO, this is losing treatment time.

B. Begin Tuan on TB disease treatment—YES

C. Consult with the public health department—NO, this is not necessary. However, the public health department must be notified.

D. Test him next year—NO, while ongoing monitoring is indicated, treatment must begin immediately, so B is the best answer.

Exhibit 3-7: Answer Details

"The presence of acid-fast-bacilli (AFB) on a sputum smear or other specimen often indicates TB disease. Acid-fast microscopy is easy and quick, but it does not confirm a diagnosis of TB because some acid-fast-bacilli are not *M. tuberculosis*. Therefore, a culture is done on all initial samples to confirm the diagnosis. (However, a positive culture is not always necessary to begin or continue treatment for TB.) A positive culture for *M. tuberculosis* confirms the diagnosis of TB disease. Culture examinations should be completed on all specimens, regardless of AFB smear results. Laboratories should report positive results on smears and cultures within 24 hours by telephone or fax to the primary health care provider and to the state or local TB control program, as required by law."

Source: CDC Division of Tuberculosis Elimination (October 28, 2011), p. 7.

Exercise 3-33: *Select all that apply*

Which of the following criteria must be met for a patient with suspected/confirmed TB to be on home isolation?

☐ Patient can speak and read English.

☒ **Patient has a stable residence at verified address.**

☒ **Patient can care for himself or herself and not require hospitalization for other medical conditions.**

☒ **Patient does not live with immunocompromised persons.**

☐ Patient has someone at home who can take care of him or her.

☒ **Patient does not live with TST-negative children.**

☒ **Environmental assessment finds the home compatible with effective isolation.**

☒ **Patient does not live in a congregate setting such as a shelter, nursing home, or single-room-occupancy hotel.**

Exercise 3-34: *Fill-in*

What are some of the other criteria for including Tuan in this program?

• **Patient is cooperative and willing to follow infection control practices.**

• **Patient is willing and competent to follow up with outpatient care with DOT.**

• **Patient signs the Home Isolation Patient Agreement.**

Exercise 3-35: *Multiple-choice question*

Tuan asks, "How did I get TB?" Warren tells Tuan that the *Mycobacterium tuberculosis* is usually transmitted by:

A. Semen and other body fluids—NO, this is not the transmission.

B. Food and water—NO, this is not the transmission.

C. Used needles—NO, this is not the transmission.

D. Airborne droplets—YES, it is airborne.

Exercise 3-36: *True or false*

The standard treatment for active TB infection is a combination therapy of four drugs: isoniazid (INH), rifampin (RIF), ethambutol (EMB), and pyrazinamide (PZA) taken daily for 9 months.

A. True

B. False

Exhibit 3-8: Answer Details

Basic TB Treatment Regimens		
Preferred Regimen	**Alternative Regimen**	**Alternative Regimen**
Initial Phase Daily INH, RIF, PZA, and EMB[a] for 56 doses (8 wk)	**Initial Phase** Daily INH, RIF, PZA, and EMB[a] for 14 doses (2 wk), then twice weekly for 12 doses (6 wk)	**Initial Phase** Thrice-weekly INH, RIF, PZA, and EMB[a] for 24 doses (8 wk)
Continuation Phase Daily INH and RIF for 126 doses (18 wk) *or* twice-weekly INH and RIF for 36 doses (18 wk)	**Continuation Phase** Twice-weekly INH and RIF for 36 doses (18 wk)	**Continuation Phase** Thrice-weekly INH and RIF for 54 doses (18 wk)

[a]Use directly observed therapy (DOT).
Source: CDC Division of Tuberculosis Elimination (June 12, 2012).

Exercise 3-37: *True or false*
Directly observed therapy (DOT) involves viewing the taking of medications to ensure compliance. This is an example of tertiary prevention.
A. True
B. False

Exercise 3-38: *Multiple-choice question*
The difference between latent TB infection and TB disease is that:
A. People with latent TB infection are not infectious, whereas people with TB disease are sometimes infectious—YES, this is the difference.
B. Only TB disease can be detected by a tuberculin skin test; latent TB infection cannot—NO, this is not true; latent will also be detected.
C. People with latent TB infection are infectious, whereas people with TB disease are not—NO, latent can also be infectious.
D. Latent TB infection is curable but TB disease is not—NO, this is not true.

Exercise 3-39: *Fill-in*
Indicate which of the following are characteristics of latent TB infection (LTBI), or TB disease, or both (B)?
LTBI	Tubercle bacilli are inactive in the body.
TB disease	Individuals are often infectious before treatment.
LTBI	Usually the chest x-ray is normal.
LTBI	Sputum smears and cultures are negative.
LTBI	Individuals do not have symptoms.

LTBI	Individuals are not infectious.
TB disease	Tubercle bacilli are active in the body.
B (Both)	The TST and QuantiFERON®-TB Gold results are usually positive.
TB Disease	Usually the chest x-ray is abnormal.
TB Disease	Sputum smears and cultures are usually positive for *M. tuberculosis*.
TB Disease	Individuals have symptoms.

Exercise 3-40: *Multiple-choice question*

The appropriate response for Maria to make is:

A. Tell Tuan that he can continue with his alternative herbal regimen along with the TB medication—NO, this is not correct.

B. Tell Tuan that there is a possibility that he can take an alternative herbal regimen as long as he continues his TB drugs, but these need to be reviewed by the doctor first—YES

C. Tell Tuan he cannot take an alternative herbal regimen and take only his TB pills—NO, this is not correct.

D. Tell Tuan to adhere to the regimen that makes him feel best—NO, this is not correct.

Exercise 3-41: *Multiple-choice question*

Maria remembers that for the purpose of the contact investigation, the end of the infectious period is determined by all of the following except:

A. Frequency and intensity of cough have improved—YES, this is not true.

B. Patient feels better—NO, this is true.

C. Patient has been receiving adequate treatment for at least 2 weeks—YES, this is not true.

D. Reduction of the grade of the AFB sputum smear or negative sputum smears—YES, this is not true.

E. A and C—NO, also D

F. A, B, and C—NO, not B

G. A, C, and D—YES, all of these

Exercise 3-42: *Multiple-choice question*

When trying to determine individuals who may have come in contact with Tuan during the infectious period, how far back should Maria ask the index patient to recall?

A. 6 months—NO, it can be different in different locales.

B. 3 months—NO, it can be different in different locales.

C. The designated time of the infectious period based on local or state standards—YES, this is true.

D. When medications were initiated—NO, this is not true.

Exercise 3-43: *Fill-in*

What is latent TB infection and how is it definitively diagnosed?

Persons with latent TB infection do not feel sick and do not have any symptoms. They are infected with *M. tuberculosis*, but do not have TB disease. The only sign of TB infection is a positive reaction to the tuberculin skin test or TB blood test. Persons with latent TB infection are not infectious and cannot spread TB infection to others (CDC, 2011, p. 2).

Exercise 3-44: *Multiple-choice question*

The standard treatment for latent TB infection is to:

A. **Give isoniazid daily for 9 months—YES, this is standard treatment.**
B. Give rifampin and isoniazid daily for 18 months—NO, standard treatment is to give isoniazid daily for 9 months
C. Closely monitor the patient's health status and then give isoniazid only if TB disease develops—NO, standard treatment is to give isoniazid daily for 9 months
D. Treat with a regimen of four drugs for 6 months—NO, one drug for 9 months
E. Treat with a regimen of three drugs for 12 months—NO, one drug, for 9 months

Exhibit 3-9: Answer Details

Latent TB Infection Treatment Regimens			
Drugs	**Duration (months)**	**Interval**	**Minimum Doses**
Isoniazid	9	Daily	270
		Twice weekly[a]	76
Isoniazid	6	Daily	180
		Twice weekly[a]	52
Isoniazid and rifapentine	3	Once weekly[a]	12
Rifampin	4	Daily	120

[a]Use directly observed therapy (DOT).
Source: CDC Division of Tuberculosis Elimination (January 20, 2012).

Exercise 3-45: *Multiple-choice question*

Which of the following statements about TB is true?

A. TB is caused by a virus—NO, TB is caused by a bacterium.
B. TB only affects the lungs—NO, TB can affect other parts of the body including the brain, kidneys, or spine.
C. **TB can be fatal—YES, if untreated, TB can be fatal.**
D. TB is highly contagious—NO, while TB is contagious, it is not easy to catch. It is more likely that you would be infected by TB by being exposed to the bacterium from someone you live with or work closely with.
E. Everyone infected with TB gets sick—NO, not everyone infected with the TB bacterium gets sick; people with the TB bacterium who do not display symptoms of illness are said to have latent TB.

Exercise 3-46: *Select all that apply*

Kim-Ly tells Maria the names and ages of the other people currently living in the home. Which members are particularly at risk for developing TB disease?

☒ **Soo-Ye, Tuan and Kim-Ly's grandmother (83 years)**

❑ Chinh-Dahn, Tuan and Kim-Ly's father (66 years)

❑ Trang, Kim-Ly's husband (48 years)

❑ Linh, Kim-Ly's daughter (22 years)

❑ Trong Tri, Linh's husband (23 years)

❑ Thomas, Kim-Ly's son (20 years)

☒ **Huu, Linh's son (5 months)**

Exercise 3-47: *Multiple-choice question*

Which of the following conditions increase the risk of developing TB disease?

A. Cardiac disease—NO, this is not a risk.

B. Kidney transplant—YES, this is the risk.

C. COPD—NO, this is not a risk.

D. Asthma—NO, this is not a risk.

Exhibit 3-10: Answer Details

The following conditions increase the risk of TB disease:

- HIV infection

- Chest x-ray findings suggestive of previous TB

- Recent TB infection (within the past 2 years)

- Prolonged therapy with corticosteroids and other immunosuppressive therapy, such as prednisone and TNF-alpha antagonists

- Silicosis

- Diabetes mellitus

- Severe kidney disease

- Certain types of cancer (e.g., leukemia, Hodgkin's disease, or cancer of the head and neck)

- Certain intestinal conditions

- Low body weight (10% or more below ideal)

- IV drug abusers (inject illegal drugs)

- Babies and young children

- Elderly people

- Those who were not treated correctly for TB in the past

Source: CDC Division of Tuberculosis Elimination (2010), p. 20.

Exercise 3-48: *Multiple-choice question*

Which of the following health conditions places a person at the highest risk of developing TB disease after becoming infected?

A. Fatigue—NO, this is not the highest risk.

B. Less than ideal body weight—NO, this is not the highest risk.

C. Pneumonia—NO, this is not the highest risk.

D. HIV infection—YES, this is the condition that immunosuppresses patients.

E. Diabetes—NO, this is not the highest risk.

Exercise 3-49: *Multiple-choice question*

HIV is a retrovirus that:

A. Attacks the immune system, destroying T-cells or CD-4 cells necessary for fighting infection—YES

B. Attacks the immune system, destroying beta cells necessary for fighting infection—NO, this is not what happens in HIV.

C. Attacks the immune system, incapacitating all cells that are necessary for fighting infection—NO, this is not what happens in HIV.

D. None of the above—NO, not all of these are true.

4

Environmental Health

Unfolding Case Study #1 ▨ Environmental Health Services

"Environmental factors influence the health of everyone," the instructor begins, "and as we have learned earlier, a major role of the public health nurse is to protect the health of *populations,* so it is reasonable to expect that the public health nurse be concerned about environmental health, right? However, it is important for you to realize that environmental health is a priority for all nurses—not just those working in community settings. In fact, Standard 16 of the American Nurses Association's (ANA) Scope and Standards of Practice addresses this very important competency." The instructor reviews the competencies associated with ANA Standard 16.

Exhibit 4-1: ANA Standard 16: Environmental Health

The registered nurse practices in an environmentally safe and healthy manner
Competencies
The registered nurse
▨ Attains knowledge of environmental health concepts, such as implantation of environmental health strategies
▨ Promotes a practice environment that reduces environmental health risks of workers and health care consumers
▨ Assesses the practice environment for factors such as sound, odor, noise, and light that negatively affect health
▨ Advocates for the judicious and appropriate use of products used in health care
▨ Communicates environmental health risks and exposure reduction strategies to health care consumers, families, colleagues, and communities
▨ Utilizes scientific evidence to determine if a product or treatment is a potential environmental threat
▨ Participates in strategies to promote healthy communities

Source: American Nurses Association (ANA) (2010).

Answers to this chapter begin on page 101.

"The environment has a great impact upon health. In fact, environmental quality has been identified as one of the 12 leading health indicators by the Healthy People 2020 initiative. Environmental health involves efforts to prevent or control environmental factors that can cause disease, injury, and disability." The instructor continues, "One important way for nurses to promote environmental health is to be aware of potential environmental health hazards. What are some environmental hazards to health?"

Exercise 4-1: *Fill-in*

List potential environmental health hazards.

_____

_____

_____

_____

eResource 4-1: To learn more about environmental hazards, the class views *Contaminated Without Consent*: http://youtu.be/jNz8yASPXoI

Exercise 4-2: *Select all that apply*

While everyone exposed to environmental hazards is at risk for developing adverse health effects and diseases, those most at risk are:

❑ Men working outdoors doing building construction

❑ Infants and small children in the community

❑ Senior citizens in a high-rise apartment building

❑ Recent immigrants living in congregate housing

❑ Hospital workers in a community hospital

Exercise 4-3: *Select all that apply*

In regard to environmental health hazards, areas for concern in homes include:

❑ Lead

❑ Radon gas

❑ Construction materials

❑ Heating methods

❑ Termite infestation

❑ Socioeconomic factors

❑ Fire safety (alarms, exits, etc.)

❑ Moisture and mold

❑ Pesticides

Answers to this chapter begin on page 101.

Exercise 4-4: *Fill-in*

What is body burden?

_____

_____

_____

 eResource 4-2: To learn more about body burden, the class views a video entitled *Chemical Body Burden*: http://youtu.be/qR8Ruqv1Zzs

eResource 4-3: To help the class better understand the concept of body burden, the instructor shows them the Environmental Working Group's 10 Americans video presentations:
- Part I: http://youtu.be/jh2p2RFAanE
- Part II: http://youtu.be/_0hSDjr-wfw
- Part III: http://youtu.be/f5Rap7RELtA

The learners are surprised to learn how pervasive chemicals are in their environment. To help the learners understand their own exposure, the instructor shows them the United States Department of Health and Human Services Household Product Database: http://householdproducts.nlm.nih.gov. She instructs them to look up a product that they use personally to see what chemicals are present in the product.

Exercise 4-5: *Fill-in*

Use the Household Product Database to look up the ingredients of a product you use regularly. List the ingredients below:

_____

_____

_____

eResource 4-4: Samantha finds an online Body Burden Assessment, which she shares with the class: http://goo.gl/Z7ENj

Amy Johnson raises her hand. "Okay, I understand that there are a lot of environmental health hazards and it seems like these hazards are everywhere. It is important for nurses to understand these risks, but how do we begin?" The instructor responds, "Certainly being aware of the risks is an important first step. As nurses, one of our primary roles is that of health education. We can do broad education such as the health hazards associated with secondhand smoke because everyone is at risk for that. But sometimes a more targeted approach is more effective. So a risk assessment is an important first step." The instructor shows the learners two assessment tools:

1. I PREPARE environmental exposure history (http://goo.gl/lm6Aq)
2. Exposure History Form

Answers to this chapter begin on page 101.

Exhibit 4-2: Exposure History Form

Part 1: Exposure Survey   Name: _____   Date: _____

Please circle the appropriate answer. Birth date: _____ Sex (circle one): Male   Female

1. Are you currently exposed to any of the following?		
metals	no	yes
dust or fibers	no	yes
chemicals	no	yes
fumes	no	yes
radiation	no	yes
biologic agents	no	yes
loud noise, vibration, extreme heat or cold	no	yes
2. Have you been exposed to any of the above in the past?	no	yes
3. Do any household members have contact with metals, dust, fibers, chemicals, fumes, radiation, or biologic agents?	no	yes

If you answered yes to any of the items above, describe your exposure in detail—how you were exposed, to what you were exposed. If you need more space, please use a separate sheet of paper.

4. Do you know the names of the metals, dusts, fibers, chemicals, fumes, or radiation that you are/were exposed to?	no	yes	If yes, list them below
5. Do you get the material on your skin or clothing?	no	yes	
6. Are your work clothes laundered at home?	no	yes	
7. Do you shower at work?	no	yes	
8. Can you smell the chemical or material you are working with?	no	yes	
9. Do you use protective equipment such as gloves, masks, respirator, or hearing protectors?	no	yes	If yes, list the protective equipment used
10. Have you been advised to use protective equipment?	no	yes	
11. Have you been instructed about the use of protective equipment?	no	yes	

Answers to this chapter begin on page 101.

12. Do you wash your hands with solvents?	no	yes			
13. Do you smoke at the workplace?	no	yes	At home?	no	yes
14. Are you exposed to secondhand tobacco smoke at the workplace?	no	yes	At home?	no	yes
15. Do you eat at the workplace?	no	yes			
16. Do you know of any co-workers experiencing similar or unusual symptoms?	no	yes			
17. Are family members experiencing similar or unusual symptoms?	no	yes			
18. Has there been a change in the health or behavior of family pets?	no	yes			
19. Do your symptoms seem to be aggravated by a specific activity?	no	yes			
20. Do your symptoms get either worse or better at work?	no	yes			
at home?	no	yes			
on weekends?	no	yes			
on vacation?	no	yes			
21. Has anything about your job changed in recent months (such as duties, procedures, overtime)?	no	yes			
22. Do you use any traditional or alternative medicines?	no	yes			

If you answered yes to any of the questions, please explain.

Answers to this chapter begin on page 101.

Part 2: Work History   Name: _____   Date: _____
A. Occupational Profile   Birth date: _____   Sex: Male Female

The following questions refer to your current or most recent job:

Job title: _____   Describe this job: _____

Type of industry: _____   _____

Name of employer: _____   _____

Date job began: _____   _____

Are you still working in this job?   no   yes

If no, when did this job end? _____

Fill in the table below listing all jobs you have worked, including short-term, seasonal, part-time employment, and military service. Begin with your most recent job. Use additional paper if necessary.

Dates of Employment	Job Title and Description of Work	Exposures*	Protective Equipment

*List the chemicals, dusts, fibers, fumes, radiation, biologic agents (i.e., molds or viruses) and physical agents (i.e., extreme heat, cold, vibration, or noise) that you were exposed to at this job.

Have you ever worked at a job or hobby in which you came in contact with any of the following by breathing, touching, or ingesting (swallowing)? If yes, please check the circle beside the name.

○ Acids	○ Chloroform	○ Mercury
○ Alcohols (industrial)	○ Chloroprene	○ Methylene chloride
○ Alkalies	○ Chromates	○ Nickel
○ Ammonia	○ Coal dust	○ PBBs
○ Arsenic	○ Dichlorobenzene	○ PCBs
○ Asbestos	○ Ethylene dibromide	○ Perchloroethylene
○ Benzene	○ Ethylene dichloride	○ Pesticides
○ Beryllium	○ Fiberglass	○ Phenol
○ Cadmium	○ Halothane	○ Phosgene
○ Carbon tetrachloride	○ Isocyanates	○ Radiation
	○ Ketones	○ Rock dust
○ Chlorinated naphthalenes	○ Lead	○ Silica powder

Answers to this chapter begin on page 101.

○ Solvents   ○ TDI or MDI   ○ Welding fumes

○ Styrene   ○ Trichloroethylene   ○ X-rays

○ Talc   ○ Trinitrotoluene   ○ Other (specify)

○ Toluene   ○ Vinyl chloride

B. Occupational Exposure Inventory   Please circle the appropriate answer.

1. Have you ever been off work for more than 1 day because of an illness related to work?	no	yes
2. Have you ever been advised to change jobs or work assignments because of any health problems or injuries?	no	yes
3. Has your work routine changed recently?	no	yes
4. Is there poor ventilation in your workplace?	no	yes

Part 3: Environmental History   Please circle the appropriate answer.

1. Do you live next to or near an industrial plant, commercial business, dump site, or nonresidential property?	no	yes
2. Which of the following do you have in your home?		

Please circle those that apply.

Air conditioner	Air purifier	Central heating (gas or oil?)	Gas stove	Electric stove
Fireplace	Wood stove	Humidifier		

3. Have you recently acquired new furniture or carpet, refinished furniture, or remodeled your home?	no	yes
4. Have you weatherized your home recently?	no	yes
5. Are pesticides or herbicides (bug or weed killers; flea and tick sprays, collars, powders, or shampoos) used in your home or garden, or on pets?	no	yes
6. Do you (or any household member) have a hobby or craft?	no	yes
7. Do you work on your car?	no	yes
8. Have you ever changed your residence because of a health problem?	no	yes
9. Does your drinking water come from a private well, city water supply, or grocery store?		
10. Approximately what year was your home built?_____		

Answers to this chapter begin on page 101.

If you answered yes to any of the questions, please explain.

Source: Agency for Toxic Substances and Disease Registry. Retrieved from http://www
.atsdr.cdc.gov/csem/cluster/docs/exposure_form.pdf

Exercise 4-6: *Fill-in*
Conduct an exposure history on an adult using Exhibit 4-2: Exposure History Form or
use the online "fillable" form: http://goo.gl/xUj8D

Exercise 4-7: *Fill-in*
Analyze the results of the exposure history you conducted, identify any priority areas
of concern, and develop a relevant client teaching plan. If no areas of concern are
identified, develop a relevant teaching plan that reflects anticipatory guidance.

_____

_____

_____

_____

_____

Exercise 4-8: *Select all that apply*
The goals of taking an exposure history include:

❑ Identifying past and present toxic exposures

❑ Enforcing Environmental Protection Agency (EPA) regulations

❑ Ending the patient's exposure to toxins

❑ Proper treatment of the patient's illness

Exercise 4-9: *Select all that apply*
Which of the following statements is true?

❑ A potential source of toxic exposure for all household members can be
hobbies.

❑ Labels required by law on household products provide sufficient
information for identifying product constituents.

❑ Most people do not know the names of the toxins that they are exposed
to on a regular basis.

❑ Family pets' health and behavior can give clues to toxic exposure in the
home.

Answers to this chapter begin on page 101.

Exercise 4-10: *Multiple-choice question*

Which of the following statements regarding the exposure history assessment are true?

    A. Exploring the chronological aspects of signs and symptoms can provide indications about the source of exposure.

    B. Knowing job titles is essential when endeavoring to ascertain toxic exposures.

    C. Employee handbooks are the best printed source of detailed information on toxic exposures.

    D. None of the above

Exercise 4-11: *True or false*

Anticipatory guidance is provided by the nurse when requested by the client or caregiver:

    A. True

    B. False

Amy conducted an exposure history assessment on her 52-year-old father, Joe Johnson, who has worked as a foreman in a shoe factory for 25 years. In doing her assessment, Amy learns that her father has two potential environmental health risks: (a) exposure to the chemical benzene and (b) loud machinery operations on the factory floor. As she prepares her teaching plan, she uses her smartphone to learn more about benzene.

 eResource 4-5: Amy opens WISER (Wireless Information System for Emergency Responders), which she had downloaded from http://wiser .nlm.nih.gov. On her device, she opens the program [Pathway: WISER → select "search known substances" → enter "benzene" into the search field → select "Medical" → read "Health Effects" and "Preventative Measures"]

Exercise 4-12: *Multiple-choice question*

Benzene is categorized as which substance type?

    A. Radiological

    B. Biological

    C. Chemical

    D. Vesicant

    E. Emollient

Exercise 4-13: *Multiple-choice question*

What is the Occupational Safety and Health Administration (OSHA) standard for benzene in the workplace?

    A. ≤0.1 ppm in 8 hours

    B. ≤1 ppm in 8 hours

    C. ≤0.01 ppm in 8 hours

    D. ≤10 ppm in 8 hours

Exercise 4-14: *Multiple-choice question*

Chronic exposure to benzene can lead to:

    A. Cardiac disease

    B. Chronic obstructive pulmonary disease

    C. Cancer

    D. Kidney failure

Answers to this chapter begin on page 101.

Exercise 4-15: *Fill-in*
What are the long-term effects of exposure to loud noises?

 eResource 4-6: To supplement her client teaching, Amy shows her father
- A presentation by Dr. Lucy Leong regarding the *Health Effects of Excessive Noise Exposure*: http://goo.gl/t5zNX
- An online Hearing Loss Simulator: http://goo.gl/qH88x

The entire class completed individual exposure histories and an individualized client education plan. "Okay, now remember community and public health is focusing on the health of *populations*. So how can we use what we learned doing the individual exposure histories and apply that to a community?"

Timothy raises his hand and says, "I guess we would start with the individual assessments, but if we notice that there are a lot of people in the community with the same problem, then we focus on that." "Yes, that is correct," says the instructor, "we look for patterns outside of the norm or standards that have been established. First, let's review. What are the core functions of public health?"

Exercise 4-16: *Select all that apply*
What are the core functions of public health?
- ❑ Assessment
- ❑ Evaluation
- ❑ Diagnosis
- ❑ Planning
- ❑ Policy development
- ❑ Advocacy
- ❑ Assurance

The instructor shows the learners a list of 10 Essential Environmental Health Services and how these relate to the core public health functions.

Exhibit 4-3: Core Functions of Public Health and How They Relate to the 10 Essential Services

Assessment
1. Monitor environmental and health status to identify and solve community environmental health problems
2. Diagnose and investigate environmental health problems and health hazards in the community

Policy Development
3. Inform, educate, and empower people about environmental health issues
4. Mobilize community partnerships and actions to identify and solve environmental health problems
5. Develop policies and plans that support individual and community environmental health efforts

Answers to this chapter begin on page 101.

Assurance

6. Enforce laws and regulations that protect environmental health and ensure safety
7. Link people to needed environmental health services and ensure the provision of environmental health services when otherwise unavailable
8. Ensure a competent environmental health workforce
9. Evaluate effectiveness, accessibility, and quality of personal and population-based environmental health services
10. Research for new insights and innovative solutions to environmental health problems

---

Source: National Center for Environmental Health (2011).

The instructor tells the class, "Clearly the first two, (a) Monitor environmental and health status to identify and solve community environmental health problems and (b) Diagnose and investigate environmental health problems and health hazards in the community, are part of *assessment*. So, let's say, for example, there is an increase of West Nile virus in a community, and while individual client education can still take place, what would be involved in a community-wide education program?"

Exercise 4-17: *Fill-in*
Design a community education program to help reduce the risk of contracting West Nile virus.

_____

_____

_____

_____

_____

_____

Unfolding Case Study #2 ▨ Michael Rowe— Lead Poisoning

Anita Rowe brings her 12-month-old son, Michael, in for a routine checkup. The nurse practitioner, Andrea Summers, asks Anita how and what Michael is eating. Anita reports, "Oh, he is a good eater. He eats solids well, lots of vegetables, and still takes his formula. I use powdered formula because it is easier to carry it home from the market and then just mix it with water from the tap." Andrea documents this and begins her initial assessment of Michael and finds the following:

- Length: 33 inches
- Weight: 24½ pounds
- Head circumference: 18¼ inches

Answers to this chapter begin on page 101.

Exercise 4-18: *Fill-in*

Plot the assessment findings on the growth chart below. How does Michael compare to the norms?

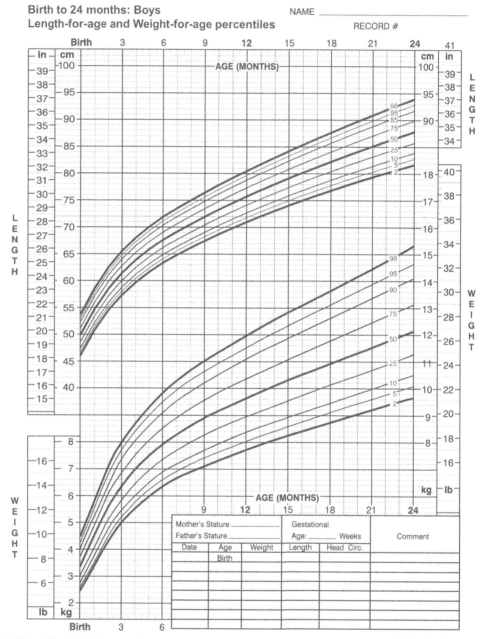

Published by the Centers for Disease Control and Prevention, November 1, 2009.
Source: WHO Child Growth Standards (http://www.who.int/childgrowth/en).

What percentile does Michael's head circumference, height, and weight fall in?

_____

Andrea reviews her findings with Anita. As Andrea completes her documentation, she notices that Anita is on Medicaid. Andrea knows that children, ages 1 to 5, who are enrolled in Medicaid are at an increased risk for elevated lead levels (*MMWR*, 2001). So she does a finger stick to test for elevated lead level.

Exercise 4-19: *Multiple-choice question*
Lead levels in children should be below:
   A. Below 5 mcg/dL
   B. Below 9 mcg/dL
   C. Between 10 and 20 mcg/dL
   D. Above 20 mcg/dL

Michael's blood lead level is 28.5 mcg/dL. Andrea also asks Anita additional questions.

Exercise 4-20: *Multiple-choice question*
What additional follow-up question(s) should be asked when screening for risk for elevated lead levels?
   A. How has Michael's appetite been?
   B. Is Michael sleeping through the night?
   C. Was your home built before 1978?
   D. Are you renting?

Andrea knows that children who have initial tests greater than 20 mcg/dL should have their home surroundings evaluated to determine the source of the lead exposure, so she asks specific questions regarding the home environment. Anita tells Andrea that the duplex she is renting for the last 6 months is older and was likely built sometime in the late 1920s. She describes it as old, but comfortable and clean. "The landlord is very nice." After further questioning, Anita admits that there is some peeling and cracking paint in the house, but doesn't understand why that is important. Andrea tells Anita that because Michael's blood lead level was above 20 mcg/dL, a home environment assessment must be conducted to determine the source of the lead and to help make the home environment safe for Michael. She goes on to explain that chipped and peeling paint in older homes is often the source of lead. "The City's Lead Poisoning Prevention Team can come and do a home environment assessment and help make your home safe."

Exercise 4-21: *Multiple-choice question*
Given the history provided by Anita and Michael's age, what might be another source of lead poisoning for Michael?
   A. Lead in the soil surrounding Anita's home
   B. Tap water in the home
   C. Fruits and vegetables from a neighborhood community garden
   D. Ceramic dishware

Answers to this chapter begin on page 101.

Andrea tells Anita that there can be other sources of lead as well.

Exercise 4-22: *Fill-in*

Besides lead in paint and old pipes, what are some other potential sources of lead?

_____

_____

_____

_____

Andrea provides some patient teaching regarding lead and why it is important to protect children from ingesting lead.

Exercise 4-23: *Fill-in*

Anita asks Andrea, "Why are children more at risk for lead poisoning?"

_____

_____

_____

 eResource 4-7: Anita is trying to understand the information that Andrea provides to her. Andrea can see that Anita is getting confused with the terminology so she gives her a booklet: *Lead Poisoning: Words to Know from A to Z*: http://goo.gl/YO4wx

Exercise 4-24: *Multiple-choice question*

Children more susceptible to lead poisoning because young children:

  A. Put things in their mouths

  B. Often have diets high in calcium

  C. Do not have mature digestive systems

  D. Crawl and play on the floors

  E. Absorb the lead more easily

  F. A, B, D, and E

  G. A, D, and E

  H. A and E

Exercise 4-25: *Multiple-choice question*

What are some of the effects of lead poisoning on children?

  A. Learning deficits

  B. High blood pressure

  C. Kidney damage

  D. A and C

  E. A, B, and C

Answers to this chapter begin on page 101.

eResource 4-8: Andrea reviews the following with Anita:

- A short video, *Lead Awareness for Parents*:
  http://youtu.be/C0HnWFrQlo4
- The Lead Safety Video: http://youtu.be/WQmrYudUloQ
- A pamphlet *Know the Facts:* A fact sheet with general lead poisoning prevention information: http://goo.gl/lDhSJ
- Additional educational materials from the CDC: http://goo.gl/QuVUg

Anita is very concerned about Michael's elevated blood lead level and asks many questions. Specifically she wants to know what she can do to help reduce his lead level. Andrea tells her that a good diet is an important first step. She explains that certain minerals are very important in preventing absorption of lead.

Exercise 4-26: *Multiple-choice question*
A deficiency of which two minerals can increase the absorption of lead?

    A. Sodium and potassium

    B. Calcium and iron

    C. Calcium and sodium

    D. Sodium and iron

Andrea goes on to explain that some foods are good sources of these important minerals, but other nutrients are also important.

Exercise 4-27: *Multiple-choice question*
What other nutrient is helpful in reducing blood lead levels?

    A. Vitamin A

    B. Vitamin B_{12}

    C. Vitamin C

    D. Vitamin E

Andrea and Anita go over a list of foods that would be good sources of these essential nutrients.

Exercise 4-28: *Matching*
Foods high in calcium, iron, and vitamin C have been identified as helpful in reducing blood lead level.

    Match the food in Column A with the nutrient (calcium, iron, or vitamin C) it has a concentration of in Column B (nutrients can be used more than once).

Column A	Column B
Milk	
Yogurt	
Low-fat cheese	

Answers to this chapter begin on page 101.

Column A	Column B
Lean red meat	
Low-fat pork	
Broccoli	
Dried beans and peas	
Raisins	
Dark green, leafy vegetables	
Low-fat cottage cheese	
Potatoes cooked in the skin	
Cabbage	
Tofu	
Strawberries	

eResource 4-9: Andrea gives Michael a coloring book that helps explain lead poisoning and how Anita's home can be made safe by the Lead Poisoning Prevention Team; the coloring book is called *Ethan's House Gets Healthier*. http://goo.gl/vB6oW

eResource 4-10: To provide additional supplemental information regarding the hazards of lead, Andrea shows Anita two short videos from Indiana State:
- Lead Paint, Lead Poisoning (Part 1): http://youtu.be/BDh46rTr-eo
- Lead Paint, Lead Poisoning (Part 2): http://youtu.be/VEJvtZqOsB8

Answers to this chapter begin on page 101.

Answers

Exercise 4-1: *Fill-in*

List potential environmental health hazards.

<u>**Environmental health hazards include:**</u>

- <u>**Dioxins**</u>
- <u>**PCBs**</u>
- <u>**Lead**</u>
- <u>**Mercury**</u>
- <u>**Air pollution**</u>
- <u>**Pesticides**</u>
- <u>**Environmental tobacco smoke**</u>
- <u>**Drinking water contamination**</u>

Exhibit 4-4: Answer Details

For more information go to Healthy People 2020:
http://healthypeople.gov/2020

Exercise 4-2: *Select all that apply*

While everyone exposed to environmental hazards is at risk for developing adverse health effects and diseases, those most at risk are:

❑ Men working outdoors doing building construction

☒ **Infants and small children in the community**

❑ Senior citizens in a high-rise apartment building

❑ Recent immigrants living in congregate housing

❑ Hospital workers in a community hospital

Exercise 4-3: *Select all that apply*

In regard to environmental health hazards, areas for concern in homes include:

☒ **Lead**

☒ **Radon gas**

☒ **Construction materials**

☒ **Heating methods**

❏ Termite infestation

❏ Socioeconomic factors

☒ **Fire safety (alarms, exits, etc.)**

☒ **Moisture and mold**

☒ **Pesticides**

Exercise 4-4: *Fill-in*

What is body burden?

Body burden is the total accumulation of chemicals within your body resulting from exposure to environmental chemicals over time.

Exercise 4-5: *Fill-in*

Use the Household Product Database to look up the ingredients of a product you use
regularly. List the ingredients below:

**Independent learning activity: using the Household Product Database to look
up the ingredients of a product you use regularly.**
Prepare to share findings in class discussion.

Exercise 4-6: *Fill-in*

Conduct an exposure history on an adult using the Exposure History Form or use
the online "fillable" form: http://goo.gl/xUj8D

Exercise 4-7: *Fill-in*

Analyze the results of the exposure history you conducted, and identify any priority
areas of concern and develop a relevant client teaching plan. If no areas of concern are
identified, develop a relevant teaching plan that reflects anticipatory guidance.

For example:
Anticipatory guidance regarding environmental exposure to lead
***Identified Risk:* Knowledge deficit related to the health risk(s) associated
with environmental exposure to lead**
Desired Outcome/Evaluation Criteria:
* **Client demonstrates improved knowledge of health risks associated with lead**
* **Client demonstrates improved knowledge of measures to reduce exposure
to lead**
* **Client takes action to reduce household exposure to lead**

Actions/Interventions:
* **Assess level of knowledge and previous learning**
* **Assess readiness to learn**
* **Provide evidence of risk (e.g., blood testing; home lead test kit)**

- **Provide educational materials:**
  - **www.cdc.gov/lead**
  - **http://goo.gl/Vb30H**
  - **www.healthfinder.gov**
- **Assist with identification of priority actions**

Exercise 4-8: *Select all that apply*
The goals of taking an exposure history include:

☒ **Identifying past and present toxic exposures**

❑ Enforcing EPA regulations

☒ **Ending the patient's exposure to toxins**

☒ **Proper treatment of the patient's illness**

Exercise 4-9: *Select all that apply*
Which of the following statements is true?

☒ **A potential source of toxic exposure for all household members can be hobbies.**

❑ Labels required by law on household products provide sufficient information for identifying product constituents.

☒ **Most people do not know the names of the toxins that they are exposed to on a regular basis.**

☒ **Family pets' health and behavior can give clues to toxic exposure in the home.**

Exercise 4-10: *Multiple-choice question*
Which of the following statements regarding the exposure history assessment are true?

A. **Exploring the chronological aspects of signs and symptoms can provide indications about the source of exposure—YES**

B. Knowing job titles is essential when endeavoring to ascertain toxic exposures—NO, this does not elicit the information needed.

C. Employee handbooks are the best printed source of detailed information on toxic exposures—NO, this describes the possible chemicals but does not pinpoint the exposure.

D. None of the above—NO, A is correct.

Exercise 4-11: *True or false*
Anticipatory guidance is provided by the nurse when requested by the client or caregiver

A. True

B. **False—YES, this is false because the nurse does not have to be asked to prove anticipatory guidance.**

Exercise 4-12: *Multiple-choice question*

Benzene is categorized as which substance type?

A. Radiological—NO

B. Biological—NO

C. Chemical—YES, benzene is a liquid chemical.

D. Vesicant—NO

E. Emollient—NO

Exercise 4-13: *Multiple-choice question*

What is the OSHA standard for benzene in the workplace?

A. ≤0.1 ppm in 8 hours—NO, this is too low.

B. ≤1 ppm in 8 hours—YES

C. ≤0.01 ppm in 8 hours—NO, this is too low.

D. ≤10 ppm in 8 hours—NO, this is excessive.

Exhibit 4-5: Answer Details

[Pathway: WISER → select "search known substances" → enter "benzene" into the search field → select "Medical" → read "OSHA Standards"]

Exercise 4-14: *Multiple-choice question*

Chronic exposure to benzene can lead to:

A. Cardiac disease—NO, there is no evidence of this in the literature.

B. Chronic obstructive pulmonary disease—NO, there is no evidence of this in the literature.

C. Cancer—YES, it attacks the body on a cellular level.

D. Kidney failure—NO, there is no evidence of this in the literature.

Exercise 4-15: *Fill-in*

What are the long-term effects of exposure to loud noises?

Exhibit 4-6: Answer Details

- Long-term exposure to excessive noise (i.e., construction, rock music, gun shot, etc.) can cause hearing loss
- Noise-induced hearing loss is one of the most common occupational illnesses. There are no visible effects, it usually develops over a long period of time, and, except in very rare cases, there is no pain
- It is a progressive loss of communication, socialization, and responsiveness to the environment. In its early stages (when hearing loss is above 2,000 Hz) it affects the ability to understand or discriminate speech. As it progresses to the lower frequencies, it begins to affect the ability to hear sounds in general
- The three main types of hearing loss are conductive, sensorineural, or a combination of the two

- **The effects of noise can be simplified into three general categories:**
  1. **Primary effects**
     - ○ **noise-induced temporary threshold shift**
     - ○ **noise-induced permanent threshold shift**
     - ○ **acoustic trauma**
     - ○ **tinnitus**
  2. **Effects on communication and performance, which may include**
     - ○ **isolation**
     - ○ **annoyance**
     - ○ **difficulty concentrating**
     - ○ **absenteeism**
     - ○ **accidents**
  3. **Other effects, which may include**
     - ○ **stress**
     - ○ **muscle tension**
     - ○ **ulcers**
     - ○ **increased blood pressure**
     - ○ **hypertension**

Exhibit 4-7: Answer Details

Occupational Safety and Health Administration (OSHA). (n.d.). http://www
.osha.gov/dts/osta/otm/noise/health_effects/index.html#effects

Exercise 4-16: *Select all that apply*

What are the core functions of public health?

☒ **Assessment**

☐ Evaluation

☐ Diagnosis

☐ Planning

☒ **Policy development**

☐ Advocacy

☒ **Assurance**

Exercise 4-17: *Fill-in*

Design a community education program to help reduce the risk of contracting West
Nile virus.

The program should involve measures to:
- **Inform, educate, and empower people about environmental health issues**
  - **CDC Information: www.cdc.gov/ncidod/dvbid/westnile**
  - **CDC: West Nile Virus TV PSA: http://youtu.be/oo-Ipp1Cx5g**
  - **West Nile Virus Presentation—Part One: http://youtu.be/ZqijoFwXgAI**
  - **West Nile Virus—Part Two: http://youtu.be/op31ontZ0sk**
- **Mobilize community partnerships and actions to identify and solve environmental health problems**
  - **Describe key stakeholders and how you will be able to mobilize the community**
  - **Efforts to eliminate mosquito reservoirs**
- **Develop (or implement) policies and plans that support individual and community environmental health efforts**
  - **Describe public health surveillance procedures and plans to protect the public's health.**

Exercise 4-18: *Fill-in*

Plot the assessment findings on the growth chart provided in the question. How does Michael compare to the norms?

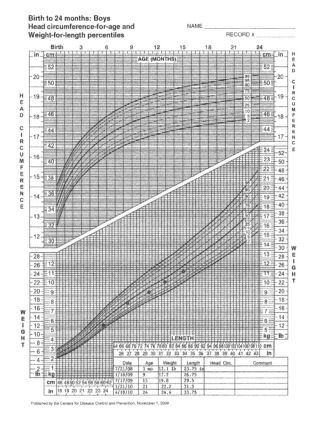

Birth to 24 months: Boys
Head circumference-for-age and
Weight-for-length percentiles

Published by the Centers for Disease Control and Prevention, November 1, 2009

What percentile does Michael's head circumference, height, and weight fall in? **At each measurement interval, Michael has consistently fallen below the 50th percentile.**

Exercise 4-19: *Multiple-choice question*

Lead levels in children should be

A. Below 5 mcg/dL—NO, this is already low.

B. Below 9 mcg/dL—YES

C. Between 10 and 20 mcg/dL—NO, this is too high.

D. Above 20 mcg/dL—NO, this is too high.

Exercise 4-20: *Multiple-choice question*

What additional follow-up question(s) should be asked when screening for risk of elevated lead levels?

A. How has Michael's appetite been?—NO, this was answered in the history.

B. Is Michael sleeping through the night?—NO, this is usually not a problem with lead poisoning.

C. Was your home built before 1978?—YES, this is significant.

D. Are you renting?—NO, this is not the issue.

Exercise 4-21: *Multiple-choice question*

Given the history provided by Anita and Michael's age, what might be another source of lead poisoning for Michael?

A. Lead in the soil surrounding Anita's home—NO, this is usually not the contaminant.

B. Tap water in the home—YES

C. Fruits and vegetables from a neighborhood community garden—NO, this is usually not the contaminant.

D. Ceramic dishware—NO, this is not the contaminant.

Exhibit 4-8: Answer Details

> Since the house is built before 1930, it is likely that the pipes contain lead. The only way to test for this is to have the water tested by a reputable lab.

Exercise 4-22: *Fill-in*

Besides lead in paint and old pipes, what are some other potential sources of lead?

- **Lead dust—caused from remodeling**
- **Soil—particularly in industrial areas and around homes built prior to 1978**
- **Artificial turf**
- **Toy jewelry**
- **Toys—paint and plastics**
- **Glazed pottery or ceramic dishware—for example, China and Mexico**
- **Imported candy—particularly from Mexico**

- **Folk medicine—used in East Indian, Indian, Middle Eastern, West Asian, and Hispanic cultures**
- **Sindoor—used as a cosmetic and in some religious ceremonies within Hindu and Sikh cultures**

Exercise 4-23: *Fill-in*

Anita asks Andrea, "Why are children more at risk for lead poisoning?"

The ability to readily absorb calcium and other nutrients is important for a child's growing body. This mechanism also increases the absorption of unwanted chemicals like lead and other heavy metals.

Exercise 4-24: *Multiple-choice question*

Children are more susceptible to lead poisoning because young children:

A. Put things in their mouths—YES
B. Often have diets high in calcium—NO, this does not affect it.
C. Do not have mature digestive systems—NO, this is not a reason.
D. Crawl and play on the floors—YES
E. Absorb the lead more easily—YES
F. A, B, D, and E—NO, not B
G. A, D, and E
H. A and E—NO, include D also

Exercise 4-25: *Multiple-choice question*

What are some of the effects of lead poisoning on children?

A. Learning deficits—YES, if the level remains high and passes the blood–brain barrier
B. High blood pressure—NO
C. Kidney damage—NO
D. A and C—NO, just A
E. A, B, and C—NO, just A

Exhibit 4-9: Answer Details

High blood pressure and kidney damage are common effects of lead poisoning among adults. Lead in a child's body can: (a) slow down growth and development, (b) damage hearing and speech, and (c) make it hard to pay attention and learn. Lead poisoning hurts the brain and nervous system. Some of the effects of lead poisoning may never go away.

Exercise 4-26: *Multiple-choice question*

A deficiency of which two minerals can increase the absorption of lead?

A. Sodium and potassium—NO, this has no effect.
B. Calcium and iron—YES
C. Calcium and sodium—NO, sodium has no effect.
D. Sodium and Iron—NO, sodium has no effect.

Exercise 4-27: *Multiple-choice question*

What other nutrient is helpful in reducing blood lead levels?

A. Vitamin A—NO, this does not lower levels of lead absorption.

B. Vitamin B_{12}—NO, this does not lower levels of lead absorption.

C. Vitamin C—YES, studies show vitamin C decreases the absorption of lead in the GI tract.

D. Vitamin E—NO, this does not lower levels of lead absorption.

Exercise 4-28: *Fill-in*

Foods high in calcium, iron, and vitamin C have been identified as helpful in reducing blood lead level.

Match the food in Column A with the nutrient (calcium, iron, or vitamin C) it has a concentration of in Column B (nutrients can be used more than once).

Column A	Column B
Milk	**Calcium**
Yogurt	**Calcium**
Low-fat cheese	**Calcium**
Lean red meat	**Iron**
Low-fat pork	**Iron**
Broccoli	**Vitamin C**
Dried beans and peas	**Iron**
Raisins	**Iron**
Dark green, leafy vegetables	**Vitamin C**
Low-fat cottage cheese	**Calcium**
Potatoes cooked in the skin	**Vitamin C**
Cabbage	**Vitamin C**
Tofu	**Calcium**
Strawberries	**Vitamin C**

5

Risk and Levels of Prevention

Unfolding Case Study #1 ■ Health Indicators and Risk

Terry Saxton and Nicole Nugent are two senior nursing students enrolled in a senior-level community and public health course. "Today," the nurse educator says, "we will learn about health indicators and the concept of risk. First, let's review the concept of health."

Exercise 5-1: *Fill-in*
What is health?

_____

_____

_____

_____

_____

Their instructor reminds the class, "Remember, our focus is on the health of *populations*. So when we look at health, we are looking at the health of the community." She goes on to tell the class that a community's health is determined by whether or not the collective health needs of the community are being met. She explains, "Health indicators such as mortality rates and disease prevalence are frequently used to describe the health of the community and serve as targets for intervention by the nurse. Healthy People 2020, a national initiative, strives to improve the health of our nation. The goal of the Healthy People initiative is to identify nationwide health improvement priorities."

Exercise 5-2: *Select all that apply*
Which of the following statements about Healthy People 2020 is true?

❏ Every 10 years, the Healthy People initiative identifies national objectives for improving the health of all Americans.

❏ The Healthy People initiative has been a national health improvement program for 20 years.

❏ The Healthy People initiative uses evidence-based practice to guide interventions.

❏ The Healthy People initiative reevaluates and revises health care priorities every 2 years.

❏ The Healthy People initiative provides a mechanism for identification of critical research, evaluation, and data collection needs.

❏ The goal of the Healthy People initiative is to increase public awareness and understanding of the determinants of health, disease, and disability and the opportunities for progress.

The instructor continues, "Another goal identified by the Healthy People 2020 initiative is to engage multiple sectors within our nation to take actions to change or strengthen policies and improve practices, with the goal of improving health." Terry raises his hand, "I notice that there are a lot of objectives identified by Healthy People 2020—over 600! It seems like a very big project." The instructor responds that a shorter subset of the objectives has been identified "as high-priority health issues to encourage focused action to address them. These are called *leading health indicators*."

Exercise 5-3: *Fill-in*
What are the leading health indicators identified by Healthy People 2020?

_____

_____

_____

_____

_____

The instructor tells the class, "These leading health indicators have been identified to help target interventions to populations who are at risk for illness. Health indicators are based upon conceptual models for what impacts health status as determined by scientific research that tracks health trends—specifically improvements in health such as increases in life expectancy, declines in mortality due to infectious diseases, and so on. These change over time."

Exercise 5-4: *Multiple-choice question*
What was the leading cause of death in the United States in the 1900s?

    A. Accidents

    B. Heart disease

    C. Pneumonia

    D. Tuberculosis

Answers to this chapter begin on page 123.

Exercise 5-5: *Multiple-choice question*

What was the leading cause of death in the United States in 2011?

    A. Violence

    B. Cancer

    C. Diabetes

    D. Heart disease

The instructor continues, "Context is important. Societal trends are continually in flux. Also, new diseases can emerge—for example, swine flu—or lifestyle behaviors like smoking or lack of exercise can have long-term impacts upon population health."

The instructor tells the class, "Often the indicator is one that has broad impact—across the life span—upon the health of a community, for example, let's consider physical inactivity." She shows the class a video about a boy named Kenyon McGriff who weighed 270 pounds by the time he was in 10th grade.

 eResource 5-1: *Meet Kenyon McGriff,* a Robert Wood Johnson Foundation's Commission to Build a Healthier America video story: http://goo.gl/ChUXR

After viewing the video, the instructor tells the class, "This is a good example of efforts to empower individuals to make informed health decisions. So let's look a little closer. First, what are the health indicators for Kenyon?"

Exercise 5-6: *Fill-in*

What were the health indicators for Kenyon?

_____

_____

_____

Exercise 5-7: *Fill-in*

What is (are) the health promotion intervention(s) for Kenyon?

_____

_____

_____

The instructor continues, "Let's explore the concept of risk from Kenyon's perspective; what does it mean to be 'at risk'?" Nicole raises her hand, "A health risk is something that increases the likelihood of disease or infirmary. For example, smoking can increase the risk of lung cancer or lung disease." "Correct, Nicole! Smoking is what we call a lifestyle behavior that can increase the likelihood of disease. What are some other lifestyle behaviors that contribute to placing an individual 'at risk'?"

Answers to this chapter begin on page 123.

Exercise 5-8: *Fill-in*
Which lifestyle behaviors place an individual at health risk?

_____

_____

_____

_____

The instructor continues, "Generally there are two types of 'risk' indicators. We've already discussed the lifestyle indicators. In addition, there are medical indicators of risk."

Exercise 5-9: *Fill-in*
What are some examples of medical indicators?

_____

_____

_____

_____

The instructor moves on to discuss levels of prevention.

Exercise 5-10: *Multiple-choice question*
Actions to protect against disease and disability are:

      A. Primary prevention

      B. Secondary prevention

      C. Tertiary prevention

      D. Both A and B

Exercise 5-11: *Select all that apply*
Primary prevention includes activities such as:

    ❑ Immunizations

    ❑ Nutrition education

    ❑ Blood sugar testing

    ❑ Application of dental sealants

    ❑ Blood pressure checks

    ❑ Water purification

    ❑ Parenting classes

Answers to this chapter begin on page 123.

Exercise 5-12: *Multiple-choice question*

Activities that attempt to prevent disease-related complications are considered:

    A. Health promotion

    B. Primary prevention

    C. Secondary prevention

    D. Tertiary prevention

Exercise 5-13: *Multiple-choice question*

Activities that strive to identify and detect disease in its earliest stages or try to prevent the spread of communicable diseases are:

    A. Health promotion

    B. Primary prevention

    C. Secondary prevention

    D. Tertiary prevention

Exercise 5-14: *Multiple-choice question*

Which of the following activities is secondary prevention?

    A. Gait training

    B. Counseling

    C. Screening

    D. Immunization

 eResource 5-2: To reinforce the class discussion regarding levels of prevention, the instructor shows the class an online tutorial: http://goo.gl/2bIsz

The instructor continues, "So, now that we have reviewed the levels of prevention, let's go back to Kenyon McGriff."

Exercise 5-15: *Fill-in*

List each of the health promotion interventions implemented for Kenyon and identify the level of prevention for each.

_____

_____

_____

_____

"Okay, class; let's look at prevention levels from a slightly different perspective now. Let's suppose that Kenyon has been diagnosed with diabetes. If we use the same interventions you have identified earlier, what would be the level of prevention?"

Answers to this chapter begin on page 123.

Exercise 5-16: *Fill-in*

If Kenyon had been diagnosed with diabetes, what would be the level of prevention?

_____

_____

_____

_____

 eResource 5-3: To supplement the value of early intervention and efforts to engage in primary prevention, the instructor shows the class a CDC-TV *A Change for Life* video: www.cdc.gov/CDCTV/ChangeForLife

Exercise 5-17: *Fill-in*

Consider Kenyon's mother, Keasha McGriff. She expresses an interest in getting healthy too. What health promotion interventions would be appropriate for her? Also, what level of prevention would each of these interventions be?

_____

_____

_____

_____

eResource 5-4: Terry is interested in learning more about the levels of prevention. He searches the web and locates an open-source textbook, *AFMC Primer on Population Health, A Virtual Textbook on Public Health Concepts for Clinicians*. Terry reads the section entitled "The Stages of Prevention": http://goo.gl/brPNE

Nicole raises her hand and asks, "You told us earlier that screening is secondary prevention because the intent is to *find people* who have the disease *before* they have clinical symptoms of disease. So then, is checking someone's blood pressure secondary prevention?" "A very good question, Nicole," replies the instructor. "Let's look closer at that so you can see the differences between the levels of prevention and what you are actually trying to accomplish with the intervention."

Exercise 5-18: *Multiple-choice question*

Checking someone's blood pressure to make sure high blood pressure is effectively controlled so as to prevent a heart attack is:

    A. Primary prevention

    B. Secondary prevention

    C. Tertiary prevention

    D. Health promotion

Answers to this chapter begin on page 123.

Exercise 5-19: *Multiple-choice question*

Checking someone's blood pressure because they have a family history of high blood pressure and stroke is:

    A. Primary prevention

    B. Secondary prevention

    C. Tertiary prevention

    D. Health promotion

Exercise 5-20: *Multiple-choice question*

Checking someone's blood pressure to make sure high blood pressure is effectively controlled so as to prevent a second heart attack is:

    A. Primary prevention

    B. Secondary prevention

    C. Tertiary prevention

    D. Health promotion

As the class continues the discussion about health risk and the story of Kenyon McGriff, Terry says, "I am really impressed that this kid was so motivated to improve his health—despite everything around him. He was 15 years old and changed the direction of his life." The instructor responds, "Yes, indeed. He certainly has reduced his risk for development of chronic diseases such as diabetes and heart disease. Part of his behavior, or rather the factors that influence *change* in his behavior, are important for health professionals to understand. This understanding can help in efforts to improve health within populations. Let's look at some models that provide a framework for better understanding of these influences."

Exercise 5-21: *Select all that apply*

Which of the following statements about the Health Belief Model is correct? Health Belief Model states that a person will take action to improve health/reduce health risk if he or she believes:

    ❑ That he or she can trust the information provided about the condition

    ❑ The consequences of the condition would be serious

    ❑ Taking action prevents the condition

    ❑ That the benefits of reducing the threat versus the cost of taking action balance out

Exercise 5-22: *Fill-in*

Consider Kenyon's actions from the perspective of the Health Belief Model. Explain his actions from the framework of the Health Belief Model.

_____

_____

_____

_____

Answers to this chapter begin on page 123.

The instructor tells the class, "Having data or information that can be easily understood by individuals is very helpful in getting a person to accept that they are at risk. Health Risk calculators can be a useful teaching tool."

 eResource 5-5: Terry does a quick search on the Internet and locates a number of free Health Calculators:

■ 10-Year CVD Risk Calculator: http://goo.gl/GHxWH

■ Framingham Coronary Risk Calculator: http://goo.gl/JxOT4

■ Health Calculators: www.healthstatus.com/calculators.html

Exercise 5-23: *Select all that apply*

The Theory of Reasoned Action is based on the following assumptions:

❑ Behavior is only influenced by intrinsic factors.

❑ Behavior is under the individual's control.

❑ People are impulsive beings.

❑ People are rational beings.

Exercise 5-24: *Select all that apply*

Social Cognitive Theory considers which of the following factors when explaining human behavior?

❑ Individual

❑ Social

❑ Cause and effect

❑ Environmental

❑ Political

The instructor concludes, "As you can see, examining health-related behavior from these models helps us understand human behavior. It can also help us predict behavior. More importantly, using these models as guides as we prepare programs and interventions helps us identify potential barriers or other things to consider prior to moving forward."

Unfolding Case Study #2 ▒ Obesity Epidemic

In class the next day, the instructor tells the class, "Yesterday, we focused our discussions on an individual, Kenyon McGriff, and his efforts to get healthy by improving his diet and increasing his physical activity. His situation is not uncommon. In fact, obesity is considered a major health problem in the United States. So let's talk some more about obesity—from a population perspective—and its impact upon our nation's health."

Answers to this chapter begin on page 123.

Exercise 5-25: *Fill-in*
How does obesity contribute to health risks?

_____

_____

_____

_____

eResource 5-6: The instructor shows the class *The Obesity Epidemic*, a video from the CDC: http://goo.gl/NbZsc

Exercise 5-26: *Fill-in*
What are factors that contribute to the problem of obesity?

_____

_____

_____

_____

eResource 5-7: Interview with Michael Pollan, in which he discusses the most important challenges and opportunities for improving our nation's food system and the role of public health: http://goo.gl/HhKPt

Exercise 5-27: *True or false*
The obesity epidemic affects children and youth equally across all socioeconomic levels.
  A. True
  B. False

The class discusses the incidence of obesity and its distribution across populations. "Is there disparity?" asks the instructor. The instructor reminds the class that looking at data like these is part of a community assessment.

Exercise 5-28: *Multiple-choice question*
Conducting a community assessment helps the nurse identify which of the following?
  A. Geographic boundaries of the community
  B. Accessibility of public transportation
  C. Community needs
  D. Housing infrastructure

eResource 5-8: The instructor tells the students to go to the CDC website and research their own community in relation to obesity and physical activity using the Youth Online Interactive Data Tables: http://goo.gl/9J6T5

Answers to this chapter begin on page 123.

The class compares their findings. To further supplement discussion regarding the problem of obesity, the instructor shows the class the following:

 eResource 5-9: The instructor shows the class:
- Video: *Children and Adolescents: The Physical Activity Guidelines in Action*: http://goo.gl/u6bSO
- CDC's podcast of an interview with Dr. Min Kyoung Song, who discusses the importance of teenagers getting enough exercise: http://goo.gl/OF2B4

"So clearly we have a serious public health problem." The instructor breaks the class up into small groups to brainstorm potential community/population focused interventions to address obesity and physical inactivity. "What are some interventions that can be done to address obesity from a community-focused or population-focused approach? Bear in mind that education will be a major part of this intervention. Be sure to consider measures to engage the entire community."

Exercise 5-29: *Multiple-choice question*
The goal of community health education is to:
> A. Change health behaviors
> B. Improve health status
> C. Provide information to make informed decisions
> D. A and B
> E. All of the above

Exercise 5-30: *Fill-in*
What are some examples of community- or population-focused interventions to address the obesity epidemic?

_____

_____

_____

_____

Unfolding Case Study #3 ▨ Noncommunicable Diseases

"Okay, class," begins the instructor. "We have learned that noncommunicable diseases (NCDs) such as heart disease and stroke, cancer, diabetes, and chronic lung disease kill more people globally than infectious diseases. As a result, these are considered the new global epidemics. Within the United States, considerable efforts are under way to address these problems." The instructor tells the class that health education and health promotion activities are essential in reducing preventable chronic disease, stating that "36 million people die each year from NCDs like heart disease and stroke, diabetes, cancer, and chronic lung disease" (WHO, 2011, p. 1).

 eResource 5-10: The instructor shows the class a series of video clips to underscore the impact of NCD upon health and introduce efforts to improve health. She points out to the class that NCDs are the leading causes of death in all countries except Africa, but Africa is expected to have the largest increase in NCDs over the next decade.

- WHO: *Unite in the fight against NCDs—Overview*: http://youtu.be/3jBsLsJvu80
- *Stop NCDs:* http://youtu.be/VCfyylZdmG0
- *Prioritizing NCDs:* http://youtu.be/Pp5RtD4zQgg
- WHO: *Unite in the fight against NCDs:* http://youtu.be/AvwX1m4LR4w
- *Unite in the fight against NCDs—September 2011:* http://youtu.be/-i_3nonEq0E

Exercise 5-31: *Multiple-choice question*
Which of the following is the cause of the greatest number of deaths globally that are attributable to noncommunicable diseases?

    A. Cancer
    B. Heart disease
    C. Diabetes
    D. Chronic lung disease

Exercise 5-32: *True or false*
Globally, deaths associated with noncommunicable disease are evenly distributed across all countries.

    A. True
    B. False

Exercise 5-33: *Select all that apply*
The primary risk factors that contribute to the majority of noncommunicable diseases include:

    ❏ Tobacco use
    ❏ High stress
    ❏ Physical inactivity
    ❏ Toxins in the environment
    ❏ Alcohol abuse
    ❏ Unhealthy diet
    ❏ IV drug abuse
    ❏ Unprotected sex

"As you can see," continues the instructor, "the primary contributing factors to NCDs are what we call *modifiable behaviors.* The incidence of NCDs can be reduced by

Answers to this chapter begin on page 123.

proactive, health protective measures. Let's go back to our earlier discussion regarding levels of prevention. Consider the risk factors of NCDs. What would be a population-focused *primary prevention* intervention for the top four risk factors?"

Exercise 5-34: *Fill-in*

List the top four risk factors for NCDs and identify a population-focused primary prevention intervention for each.

Risk Factor	Population-Focused Primary Prevention

The instructor continues, "Primary prevention is important but early identification and intervention before serious disease occurs are also priorities. Remember, secondary prevention seeks to find individuals *before* they exhibit clinical symptoms of disease."

Exercise 5-35: *Fill-in*

List the top four risk factors for NCDs and identify a population-focused secondary prevention intervention for each.

Risk Factor	Population-Focused Secondary Prevention

Answers to this chapter begin on page 123.

Answers

Exercise 5-1: *Fill-in*

What is health?

Health is defined as:

"... the state of complete physical, mental and social well-being and not merely the absence of disease or infirmity" (WHO, 1946) and the "extent to which an individual or group is able to realize aspirations and satisfy needs, and to change or cope with the environment. Health is a resource for everyday life, not the objective of living; it is a positive concept, emphasizing social and personal resources as well as physical capabilities" (WHO, 1984).

Exercise 5-2: *Select all that apply*

Which of the following statements about Healthy People 2020 is true?

❑ Every 10 years, the Healthy People initiative identifies national objectives for improving the health of all Americans.

❑ The Healthy People initiative has been a national health improvement program for 20 years.

☒ **The Healthy People initiative uses evidence-based practice to guide interventions.**

❑ The Healthy People initiative reevaluates and revises health care priorities every 2 years.

☒ **The Healthy People initiative provides a mechanism for identification of critical research, evaluation, and data collection needs.**

☒ **The goal of the Healthy People initiative is to increase public awareness and understanding of the determinants of health, disease, and disability and the opportunities for progress.**

Exercise 5-3: *Fill-in*

What are the leading health indicators identified by Healthy People 2020?

1. **Access to health services**
2. **Clinical preventive services**
3. **Environmental quality**
4. **Injury and violence**
5. **Maternal, infant, and child health**

6. **Mental health**
7. **Nutrition, physical activity, and obesity**
8. **Oral health**
9. **Reproductive and sexual health**
10. **Social determinants**
11. **Substance abuse**
12. **Tobacco**

Exercise 5-4: *Multiple-choice question*
What was the leading cause of death in the United States in the 1900s?
A. Accidents—NO, this increased with the use of motor vehicles.
B. Heart disease—NO, dietary habits were healthier.
C. Pneumonia—YES, lack of antibiotics
D. Tuberculosis—NO, not in the United States, but in other places in the world this was prevalent

Exercise 5-5: *Multiple-choice question*
What was the leading cause of death in the United States in 2011?
A. Violence—NO, although this is on the rise
B. Cancer—NO, although cancer claims many lives
C. Diabetes—NO, but again this is on the rise
D. Heart disease—YES, due to sedentary lifestyles and dietary changes

Exercise 5-6: *Fill-in*
What were the health indicators for Kenyon?
Nutrition, physical activity, and obesity

- **Overweight, 270 pounds**
- **Poor diet**
- **Sedentary lifestyle (no exercise)**

Environmental: Exposure to secondhand smoke (mother is a heavy smoker)

Social determinants

- **Lives in urban area with limited access to recreation**
- **Low income**
- **Minority**

Contributing factors

- **Dark neck → increased risk for diabetes**
- **Family history of diabetes (mother, aunt, and grandmother) and heart trouble (grandfather died of heart disease)**

Exercise 5-7: *Fill-in*

What is (are) the health promotion intervention(s) for Kenyon?

1. **General healthy lifestyle education**
2. **Physical activity**
3. **Nutrition education**
4. **Diet modification**
5. **Environmental modification—reduction of exposure to secondhand smoke**

Exercise 5-8: *Fill-in*

Which lifestyle behaviors place an individual at health risk?

Lifestyle "at risk" indicators include:

- **Physical activity**
- **Tobacco use**
- **Dietary fat intake**
- **Fruit/vegetable intake**
- **Stress**
- **Alcohol intake**
- **Seat belt use**

Exercise 5-9: *Fill-in*

What are some examples of medical indicators?

Medical indicators include:

- **Total cholesterol–high-density lipoprotein ratio**
- **Blood pressure**
- **Blood glucose**
- **Weight**
- **Triglycerides**

Exercise 5-10: *Multiple-choice question*

Actions to protect against disease and disability are:

A. **Primary prevention—YES**

B. Secondary prevention—NO, this is after a condition is diagnosed.

C. Tertiary prevention—NO, this is trying to control a known condition.

D. Both A and B—NO

Exercise 5-11: *Select all that apply*

Primary prevention includes activities such as:

☒ **Immunizations**

☒ **Nutrition education**

❏ Blood sugar testing

☒ **Application of dental sealants**

❏ Blood pressure checks

☒ **Water purification**

☒ **Parenting classes**

Exhibit 5-1: Answer Details

Primary prevention seeks to promote health and *prevent* disease from occurring.

Exercise 5-12: *Multiple-choice question*
Activities that attempt to prevent disease-related complications are considered:
  A. Health promotion—NO, this is preventing disease itself.
  B. Primary prevention—NO, this is intervening in the early stages.
  C. Secondary prevention—NO, this is treating the primary disease.
  D. **Tertiary prevention—YES**

Exhibit 5-2: Answer Details

Tertiary prevention goal is to interrupt the progress of the disease, reduce the amount of disability, and begin rehabilitation, for example, diabetes classes, Narcotics Anonymous.

Exercise 5-13: *Multiple-choice question*
Activities that strive to identify and detect disease in its earliest stages or try to prevent the spread of communicable diseases are:
  A. Health promotion—NO, this is improving lifestyle to decrease risk factors that are modifiable.
  B. Primary prevention—NO, this is early identification.
  C. **Secondary prevention—YES**
  D. Tertiary prevention—NO, this is dealing with complications.

Exhibit 5-3: Answer Details

Secondary prevention includes interventions designed to increase the likelihood that a person with a disease will be diagnosed early enough so that the treatment may result in a cure. Secondary prevention goal is to detect the disease in early stages *before* signs and symptoms become apparent to make an early diagnosis and begin treatment. Examples include screening and education of "at risk" populations. See Exhibits 5-4 and 5-5 for more information.

Exhibit 5-4: Levels of Prevention

Primary Prevention

Interventions directed at preventing problem(s) from ever occurring

Prevention during the prepathogenesis or susceptibility stage. The purpose of primary prevention is to reduce risk and promote health. Examples: Immunizations, water purification, sewage treatment, nutrition education, smoking cessation, healthy lifestyles, and so forth

Secondary Prevention

Interventions directed at early recognition and diagnosis of problems

Early detection and prompt treatment of the disease, generally during the presymptomatic stage. Examples: Screening for diseases (e.g., glaucoma, hypertension, diabetes, cervical cancer, prostate cancer, etc.)

Tertiary Prevention

Palliation and prevention of further deterioration

Activities to reduce the effects of diseases that have already occurred. These activities take place during the clinical stages of the disease. Examples: Physical therapy and rehabilitation of stroke victims, support services for the disabled, and so forth

Source: Montana Public Health Department (n.d.), p. 8.

Exhibit 5-5: Public Health Nursing Services by Levels of Prevention

Primary Prevention	Secondary Prevention	Tertiary Prevention
Coalition-building to conduct a community assessment	Health screening, case finding, and referral (e.g., hypertension and communicable diseases)	Case management for disabled children
Partnering with community agencies to plan courses of action for needs identified in the assessment	Health screening, case finding, and referral for alcohol and drug abuse and other mental health problems	Case management for disabled adults
Prenatal care clinics		Case management for frail, elderly individuals
Family planning clinics	Health screening, case finding, and referral for children with developmental delays and disabilities	Home health care
Health education for health promotion and risk reduction		Geriatric evaluations before institutional placement
		Adult medical day care

(continued)

**Exhibit 5-5: Public Health Nursing Services
by Levels of Prevention (*continued*)**

Primary Prevention	Secondary Prevention	Tertiary Prevention
Identification of those at risk for communicable diseases	Outreach during home visits and at work sites and schools to identify targeted populations, such as pregnant women, adolescents, and chronically ill and disabled persons	
Identification of those at risk for alcohol and drug abuse and other mental health problems		
Immunizations (education campaigns and clinics)	Contact investigation for communicable diseases	
Anticipatory guidance for parents regarding child care and parenting	Clinics for sexually transmitted diseases	
Safety and environmental education	Clinics for tuberculosis	
Home visits for health promotion for pregnant women, new parents, and frail, elderly individuals	Treatment for specific illnesses (e.g., medications for sexually transmitted diseases based on medical orders and treatment protocols)	
School health promotion, especially regarding substance abuse, pregnancy, and violence prevention	Primary care clinics	
	Clinics for the homeless	
Worker health promotion programs	Environmental surveillance	
Inspection and licensing (nursing homes and day-care centers)		

Source: Maurer and Smith (2009), pp. 753–754.

Exercise 5-14: *Multiple-choice question*

Which of the following activities are secondary prevention?

A. Gait training—NO, this is tertiary.

B. Counseling—NO, this is tertiary.

C. Screening—YES, this is secondary.

D. Immunization—NO, this is primary.

Exercise 5-15: *Fill-in*

List each of the health promotion interventions implemented for Kenyon and identify the level of prevention for each.

1. **General healthy lifestyle education—Primary prevention**

2. **Physical activity—Primary prevention**

3. **Nutrition education—Primary prevention**

4. **Diet modification—Primary prevention**

5. **Environmental modification—reduction of exposure to second-hand smoke— Primary prevention**

Exhibit 5-6: Note

Since Kenyon has not exhibited any signs or symptoms of disease, all of these efforts are considered primary prevention efforts.

Exercise 5-16: *Fill-in*

If Kenyon had been diagnosed with diabetes, what would be the level of prevention?

1. **General healthy lifestyle education—Primary prevention**

2. **Diabetes education—Tertiary prevention**

   a. **Physical activity—Tertiary prevention**

   b. **Nutrition education—Tertiary prevention**

   c. **Diet modification—Tertiary prevention**

3. **Environmental modification—reduction of exposure to secondhand smoke— Primary prevention (remember, there is no evidence of disease, so it remains primary)**

Exhibit 5-7: Note

Remember, since Kenyon has not exhibited any signs or symptoms of disease, all of these efforts are considered primary prevention efforts.

Exercise 5-17: *Fill-in*

Consider Kenyon's mother, Keasha McGriff. She expresses an interest in getting healthy too. What health promotion interventions would be appropriate for her? Also, what level of prevention would each of these interventions be?

1. **General healthy lifestyle education—Primary prevention**

2. **Smoking cessation—Secondary prevention**

3. **Diabetes education (general self-care, management, etc.)—Tertiary prevention**

4. **Diet and nutrition education (diabetic diet)—Tertiary prevention**

5. **Physical activity—Primary prevention**

6. **Stress management—Primary prevention**

Exercise 5-18: *Multiple-choice question*

Checking someone's blood pressure to make sure high blood pressure is effectively controlled so as to prevent a heart attack is:

A. Primary prevention—YES, this is decreasing risks of a myocardial infarction (MI), not preventing the hypertension.

B. Secondary prevention—NO, this is screening for an abnormal heart function.

C. Tertiary prevention—NO, this is intervening in an MI.

D. Health promotion—NO, this is part of primary care.

Exercise 5-19: *Multiple-choice question*

Checking someone's blood pressure because they have a family history of high blood pressure and stroke is:

A. Primary prevention—NO, the risk factors already exist and are nonmodifiable.

B. Secondary prevention—YES, this is screening.

C. Tertiary prevention—NO, this would mean the patient is already hypertensive.

D. Health promotion—NO, this is primary care.

Exercise 5-20: *Multiple-choice question*

Checking someone's blood pressure to make sure high blood pressure is effectively controlled so as to prevent a second heart attack is:

A. Primary prevention—NO, it is too late to modify behavior.

B. Secondary prevention—NO, it is more than screening and prevention.

C. Tertiary prevention—YES, it is controlling the condition.

D. Health promotion—NO, this is part of primary care.

Exercise 5-21: *Select all that apply*

Which of the following statements about the Health Belief Model is correct? Health Belief Model states that a person will take action to improve health/reduce health risk if he or she believes:

❑ A person will take action if he or she trusts the information provided about the condition.

☒ **The consequences of the condition would be serious.**

☒ **Taking action prevents the condition.**

❑ A person will take action if the benefits of reducing the threat versus the cost of taking action balance out.

Exhibit 5-8: Answer Details

The Health Belief Model is based upon the assumption that people will take corrective action to improve their health and reduce risk if they believe that:

- they are susceptible/vulnerable to the disease/condition

- getting the disease/condition would be a serious consequence

- they are capable of taking action and that action can prevent the disease/condition

- the benefits of reducing the risk of the disease/condition outweigh the costs of taking preventive action

Exercise 5-22: *Fill-in*

Consider Kenyon's actions from the perspective of the Health Belief Model. Explain his actions from the framework of the Health Belief Model. Remember that the Health Belief Model is based upon the assumption that people will take corrective action to improve their health and reduce risk if they believe that:

Table 5-1

1. They are susceptible or vulnerable to the disease/condition	Kenyon's doctor was very frank about assessment; Kenyon has a strong family history of obesity-related disease (diabetes, heart disease)
2. Getting the disease/condition would be a serious consequence	Kenyon was told by the doctor that he "... could expect a lifetime of back pain, insulin shots, and heart attacks"
3. They are capable of taking action and that action can prevent the disease/condition	Kenyon believed that he could change his health by changing his behaviors: Eating better (gave up sugary drinks and greasy fried foods) and exercising (running club) would improve his health
4. The benefits of reducing the risk of the disease/condition outweigh the costs of taking preventive action	• "I told myself I was going to stop being unhealthy" • Able to run greater distances over time • Lost some friends but still kept it up • Realized the "path to good health was an obstacle course in which money, education, and one's environment can prove to be especially challenging"

Exercise 5-23: *Select all that apply*

The Theory of Reasoned Action is based on the following assumptions:

❑ Behavior is only influenced by intrinsic factors.

☒ **Behavior is under the individual's control.**

❑ People are impulsive beings.

☒ **People are rational beings.**

Exercise 5-24: *Select all that apply*

Social Cognitive Theory considers which of the following factors when explaining human behavior?

☒ **Individual**

☒ **Social**

❑ Cause and effect

☒ **Environmental**

❑ Political

Exhibit 5-9: Answer Details

> Social Cognitive Theory "states that there is a continuous, dynamic interaction between the individual, the environment, and behavior. Thus, a change in one of these factors impacts on the other two."

Source: Redding, Rossi, Rossi, Velicer, and Prochaska (2000), p. 185.

Exercise 5-25: *Fill-in*

How does obesity contribute to health risks?

Obesity is directly linked to the following:

• **Type 2 diabetes**

• **Cardiovascular disease**

• **Breast cancer**

• **Colon cancer**

• **Gallbladder disease**

• **High blood pressure**

Exercise 5-26: *Fill-in*

What are factors that contribute to the problem of obesity?

• **Processed food**

• **Access to healthy foods**

• **Technology**

• **Community environment**

• **Sedentary lifestyles**

Exercise 5-27: *True or false*

The obesity epidemic affects children and youth equally across all socioeconomic levels.

A. True

B. False

Exhibit 5-10: Answer Details

> "Overweight and obesity in childhood have emerged during the past five years as among **the most pressing public health issues for children and youth**. Nearly a third (31.6 percent) of all children ages 10–17 are overweight or obese . . . . In addition to the increase in obesity, these data reveal that the **concentration of the epidemic among poor and minority children has increased** since 2003 . . . rates of overweight and obesity were greatest among poor, Black, Hispanic, and publicly insured children."

Source: Bethell, Simpson, Stumbo, Carle, and Gombojav (2010), p. 354.

Exercise 5-28: *Multiple-choice question*

Conducting a community assessment helps the nurse identify which of the following?

A. Geographic boundaries of the community—NO, this does not define the needs of the community.

B. Accessibility of public transportation—NO, this is part of it but not the main purpose.

C. Community needs—YES

D. Housing infrastructure—NO, this is part of it but not the main purpose.

Exercise 5-29: *Multiple-choice question*

The goal of community health education is to:

A. Change health behaviors—YES

B. Improve health status—YES

C. Provide information to make informed decisions—YES

D. A and B—NO, also C

E. All of the above—YES, they are all goals and need to be considered.

Exercise 5-30: *Fill-in*

What are some examples of community- or population-focused interventions to address the obesity epidemic?

> **To identify a variety of community- or population-focused interventions to address the obesity epidemic, please view these videos that showcase community-based programs to address childhood obesity:**
>
> - CDC-TV video, *Making Health Easier: Healthy Changes Start in Preschool:* www.cdc.gov/CDCTV/ChildObese
> - *100 Citizens: Role Model for the Future:* http://youtu.be/o7FIwQNKvH8
> - *Let's Move—Tools and Resources:* www.letsmove.gov/resources

Exercise 5-31: *Multiple-choice question*

Which of the following is the cause of the greatest number of deaths globally that are attributable to noncommunicable diseases?

A. Cancer—NO, this is not the greatest cause, although it kills many people globally.

B. Heart disease—YES

C. Diabetes—NO, this is not the greatest cause, although it kills many people globally.

D. Chronic lung disease—NO, this is not the greatest cause, although it kills many people globally.

Exercise 5-32: *True or false*

Globally, deaths associated with noncommunicable diseases are evenly distributed across all countries.

A. True

B. False—NO, nearly 80% of NCD deaths—29 million—occur in low- and middle-income countries (WHO, 2011).

Exercise 5-33: *Select all that apply*

The primary risk factors that contribute to the majority of noncommunicable diseases include:

☒ **Tobacco use**

☐ High stress

☒ **Physical inactivity**

☐ Toxins in the environment

☒ **Alcohol abuse**

☒ **Unhealthy diet**

☐ IV drug abuse

☐ Unprotected sex

Exhibit 5-11: Answer Details

Primary risk factors: tobacco use, physical inactivity, the harmful use of alcohol and unhealthy diets

Source: WHO (2011).

Exercise 5-34: *Fill-in*

List the top four risk factors for NCDs and identify a population-focused primary prevention intervention for each.

Table 5-2

Risk Factor	Population-Focused Primary Prevention
1. Tobacco use	Smoking prevention programs; public policy to discourage smoking (no sales to minors; taxes; no smoking areas; no advertising; limited placement of cigarette vending machines, etc.)
2. Physical inactivity	School fitness programs designed to get children physically active; public spaces to encourage physical activity; bike and walk paths; incentives to bike to work
3. Unhealthy diet	Health education; improved access to healthy foods; community gardens; school-based programs that get families involved; public policies to restrict junk food at schools
4. Alcohol abuse	Underage drinking prevention programs; early intervention (no sales to minors; taxes; etc.)

Exercise 5-35: *Fill-in*

List the top four risk factors for NCDs and identify a population-focused secondary prevention intervention for each.

Table 5-3

Risk Factor	Population-Focused Primary Prevention
1. Tobacco use	Smoking cessation programs (can be primary or secondary depending upon how long the individual has been a smoker)
2. Physical inactivity	In addition to school fitness programs designed to get children physically active, public spaces to encourage physical activity; bike and walk paths; incentives to bike to work; also have insurance incentives; free or subsidized health club memberships; employer incentives
3. Unhealthy diet	Health education; health screening using tools that demonstrate level of risk (e.g., cardiovascular disease risk tool; blood pressure screening; stroke screening, etc.); diet counseling; improved access to healthy foods; community gardens
4. Alcohol abuse	Underage drinking cessation programs (Alcoholic Anonymous programs)

Exhibit 5-12: Note

Primary-level interventions and secondary-level interventions are frequently similar, but the focus is different—prevention versus early intervention.

6

Vulnerable Populations

Unfolding Case Study #1 ▨ Being Vulnerable in the United States

"The United States is considered one of the most advanced and rich countries in the world, yet we also have some of the greatest inequities when it comes to health," the nurse educator told the class. "Today, we will explore the concept of vulnerability and factors that contribute to being vulnerable."

Exercise 6-1: *Fill-in*
What does it mean to be vulnerable? Provide an example of a vulnerable patient.

_____

_____

_____

_____

Exercise 6-2: *Fill-in*
Define vulnerable populations.

_____

_____

_____

_____

Exercise 6-3: *Fill-in*
Which populations are considered vulnerable populations?

_____

_____

_____

_____

Exercise 6-4: *Select all that apply*

Vulnerable populations frequently have less control over their health due to:

❑ Socioeconomic factors

❑ Income

❑ Education

❑ Access issues

❑ Health beliefs

❑ Disenfranchisement

The instructor tells the class that vulnerable populations are a focus of public health because the health of populations has implications for public health and its core functions, especially that of assurance, which strives to provide essential personal health services for those who would otherwise not receive it. "Public health efforts strive to break the cycle of vulnerability because without accomplishing that, it is difficult to change health behavior," states the instructor.

Figure 6-1: Cycle of Vulnerability

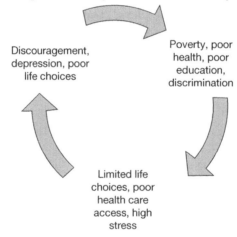

Discouragement, depression, poor life choices

Poverty, poor health, poor education, discrimination

Limited life choices, poor health care access, high stress

Exercise 6-5: *Fill-in*

What factors contribute to vulnerability?

_____

_____

_____

_____

The instructor tells the class, "Remember, the focus of community and public health is upon the health of populations. So it makes sense that vulnerable populations are a concern . . . certainly because of the characteristic of vulnerability

Answers to this chapter begin on page 154.

and the health risks associated with that. But there is more to consider . . . there are broader implications. What would be the broader public health implications associated with the health of vulnerable populations?"

Exercise 6-6: *Fill-in*

What are the broader public health implications associated with the health of vulnerable populations?

_____

_____

_____

Exercise 6-7: *Multiple-choice question*

An example of an individual from a vulnerable population is:

    A. Person with asthma who lives next to a factory that manufactures tires

    B. Person with COPD who lives next to a pharmacy

    C. Person with a cold who is not taking antibiotics

    D. Person with a 3-cm area of erythema 24 hours after a PPD test

Exercise 6-8: Multiple-choice question

Which of the following best reflects the definition of a vulnerable population?

    A. The homeless population in a large city

    B. Groups that are susceptible to certain communicable diseases

    C. Groups that have an increased risk of developing adverse health outcome

    D. Groups that live in low-income housing

Exercise 6-9: *Multiple-choice question*

All of the following are examples of a vulnerable population except

    A. Severely mentally ill

    B. Migrant workers

    C. Impoverished population

    D. Nursing students

"Poverty," said the instructor, "is one of the major factors that contribute to vulnerability. Let's look at poverty more closely. What is poverty?"

Exercise 6-10: *Fill-in*

Define poverty:

_____

_____

_____

"Let's look more closely at the level of poverty in the United States. Let's compare the levels of poverty within various states."

Answers to this chapter begin on page 154.

eResource 6-1: The instructor shows the class the Kaiser Foundation's State Health Database: [Pathway: www.statehealthfacts.org → select "Demographics and the Economy" → select "Compare: Two Locations"]

Exercise 6-11: *Fill-in*

What is the federal poverty level? How is it determined?

_____

_____

_____

eResource 6-2: To view the current Federal Poverty Income Guidelines, go to: http://goo.gl/n2VhO or http://goo.gl/Jiabq

eResource 6-3: To download the U.S. Census Bureau's mobile app, go to: www.census.gov/mobile

Exercise 6-12: *Multiple-choice question*

_____ is a concept that implies that some people are worthy to have a roof over their heads and others not.

    A. Maleficence

    B. Distributive justice

    C. Creative justice

    D. Fair and Equal Division of Resource Act

The instructor continues, "Let's review the concept of *risk*. Remember there are many factors that affect health status. These factors, when compounded, as is the case for vulnerable populations, increase the likelihood of illness or poor health outcomes."

Figure 6-2: Factors That Affect Health Status

Values and beliefs • Environment • Economic status • Access to services • Housing • Psychological impact of poverty • Mental health • Occupation/employment status • Age • Gender • Race/ethnicity • Policy • Lifestyle behaviors • Genetic heredity • Social supports • Culture → **Health status**

Answers to this chapter begin on page 154.

"Some people have a higher probability of illness than others do. Consider this from an epidemiological perspective. In the epidemiological triangle, the agent, host, and environment interact to produce illness or poor health."

Figure 6-3: Epidemiological Triangle—Interactions That Produce Poor Health or Illness

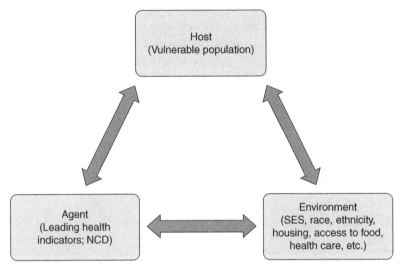

e **eResource 6-4:** To help the class understand the socioeconomic factors that influence vulnerability and how the cycle is perpetuated, the instructor shows the class a series of video excerpts from the documentary *Unnatural Causes: Is Inequality Making Us Sick?*
- *In Sickness and Wealth*: http://goo.gl/K2uw6
- *There's No Such Thing as Small Stuff: Being Poor in Louisville*: http://goo.gl/0Pne5
- *Growing Wealth Divide Is Bad for Health*: http://goo.gl/SXEGS
- *Living in Disadvantaged Neighborhoods Is Bad for Your Health*: http://goo.gl/iIg6B

"Clearly, these videos show how poverty can affect health." The instructor continues, "*but*, it is important to note that not everyone who is at risk will develop the illness. Why is that?"

Exercise 6-13: *Fill-in*
What is resiliency?

_____

_____

Answers to this chapter begin on page 154.

Exercise 6-14: *Fill-in*

What is the Latino Paradox?

_____

_____

_____

_____

"Okay, now. Let's review. What do resiliency and the Latino Paradox tell us?" The instructor asks the class. Gerald raises his hand. "That we need to be aware that people are different and not to stereotype individuals or groups." "That's correct, Gerald," the instructor replies. "The concept of health and factors contributing to health and health outcomes are very complex. It is important that we keep in mind the value of social influences—such as community and family, cultural values—and use these strengths to support positive health outcomes." The instructor tells the class, "The poverty rate has risen disproportionately among vulnerable populations. There are factors that have been identified that can help break the cycle of poverty. First, let's review the overarching goals of Healthy People 2020."

Exercise 6-15: *Fill-in*

What are the overarching goals of Healthy People 2020?

1. _____

2. _____

3. _____

4. _____

"As we have seen," the instructor continues, "a key factor to consider in efforts to meet these overarching goals is the matter of poverty. Poverty is interwoven in all of this. If poverty can be addressed, there can be significant gains in health status."

Exhibit 6-1: Health Effect of Poverty

Increased mortality and morbidity due to:	Reduced access to care due to:
• Race	• Lack of transportation
• Gender (women)	• Inability to leave jobs for appointments
• Poor housing	• Lack of health insurance
• Racism	• No "sick time"
• Neighborhood violence	• Receiving unequal care
• Poverty stressors	• Receiving inconsistent care
• Educational and job status	• Treatment without health promotion
• Learned helplessness	• Limited health care providers/health resources

Answers to this chapter begin on page 154.

Exercise 6-16: *Fill-in*
How does poverty influence vulnerability?

_____

_____

eResource 6-5: To see the influence of education on health status, go to: Education and Health Calculator: http://goo.gl/6tNAW

Exercise 6-17: *Multiple-choice question*
Poverty is defined as:
A. Having insufficient financial resources to meet basic living expenses for food, clothing, shelter, transportation, and health care
B. A family of four with income less than $32,000
C. A homeless man that goes to the St. John's Hospice daily for lunch
D. Having insufficient financial resources to meet the mortgage payments on a monthly basis

"Okay, now that we have the concept of vulnerability down," said the instructor, "let's apply what we have learned about vulnerability to a couple of realistic situations."

eResource 6-6: The instructor shows the class a segment from ABC's *20/20* with Diane Sawyer, "Waiting on the World to Change—Children in Poverty: The Hopes and Hurdles of Children in Poverty." The segment is about Billy, an adolescent who lives in Camden, New Jersey: http://goo.gl/5suYe

Exercise 6-18: *Fill-in*
What factors make Billy vulnerable?

_____

_____

_____

Exercise 6-19: *Fill-in*
What are the issues/concerns for Billy?

_____

_____

_____

_____

_____

Answers to this chapter begin on page 154.

Exercise 6-20: *Fill-in*

Identify interventions for Billy at the primary, secondary, and tertiary levels for one of the issues/concerns identified in the previous exercise.

1. _____
2. _____
3. _____

ⓔ   **eResource 6-7:** The instructor shows the class a second video, *Meet the Elkins' Family*: http://goo.gl/KFm9v

Exercise 6-21: *Fill-in*

What factors make the Elkins' family vulnerable?

_____

_____

_____

_____

Exercise 6-22: *Fill-in*

What are the issues/concerns for the Elkins' family?

_____

_____

_____

_____

_____

Exercise 6-23: *Fill-in*

Identify interventions for the Elkins' family at the primary, secondary, and tertiary levels for one of the issues/concerns identified in the previous exercise.

1. _____
2. _____
3. _____

Answers to this chapter begin on page 154.

Unfolding Case Study #2 Sexual Activity and Teenage Pregnancy

Stephanie Rosen is a school nurse in the middle school of a large urban school district. The school's population is diverse; however, the majority are African American or Black (52%) and Hispanic (35%). She knows that adolescents are a vulnerable population and are at risk for poor health outcomes related to a variety of factors including risky behavior, impulsivity, unprotected sex, and violence.

eResource 6-8: To better understand adolescent behavior and the typical impulsivity observed in this population, Stephanie views a video presentation by neuroscientist Dr. Sarah-Jayne Blackmore, *The Mysterious Workings of the Adolescent Brain*: http://on.ted.com/Blakemore

Exercise 6-24: *Multiple-choice question*
Stephanie is working with teens in a high school life skills class. They are discussing attitudes and feelings about smoking; the nurse uses role playing as a teaching tool. This is an example of which of the following domains of learning?

    A. Cognitive

    B. Psychomotor

    C. Affective

    D. Teaching

Stephanie knows that while there has been a decrease in teen pregnancy rates over the last 10 years, the United States still has a pregnancy rate that is "one of the highest in the developed world" (Kost & Henshaw, 2012; Singh & Darroch, 2000).

Figure 6-4: Teen Pregnancy Rates, 2000–2010

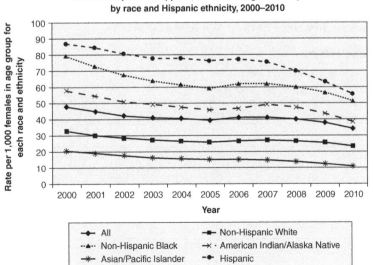

Birth rates (live births) per 1,000 females aged 15–19 years, by race and Hispanic ethnicity, 2000–2010

Source: Hamilton, Martin, and Ventura (2011).

Answers to this chapter begin on page 154.

Figure 6-5: Teen Pregnancy Rates in Industrialized Countries

U.S. Teen births highest of all industrialized countries

Country	Rate
Bulgaria	42
U.S.	39
Turkey	39
Romania	31
U.K.	24
Ireland	16
Israel	14
Canada	13
Norway	9
Sweden	8
Germany	8
France	7
Italy	5
Japan	5
Netherlands	4

Live Births per 1,000 females age 15–19 years

Source: International data: United Nations (2008).
U.S. data: Hamilton, Martin, and Ventura (2010).

She also knows that in the United States a key concern among health care professionals is teenage pregnancy. Public health efforts to address teenage pregnancy have been successful, due in part to improved contraceptive use and increased proportions of teens choosing to delay sexual activity. However, Stephanie also knows that pregnancy rates for African American teens and Hispanic teens are two to three times higher than in their White counterparts.

Exercise 6-25: *Fill-in*

Teen pregnancy is a concern because:

_____

_____

_____

_____

Exercise 6-26: *Fill-in*

Factors that contribute to teenage pregnancy include:

_____

_____

_____

Answers to this chapter begin on page 154.

e **eResource 6-9:** To better understand her role as a health care provider, Stephanie listens to two CDC presentations:

- Dr. Wanda Barfield, Director of CDC's Division of Reproductive Health, where she discusses the responsibility of health care providers in *Teen Pregnancy and Reproductive Health*: http://goo.gl/peiXV
- *A Message to Health Care Professionals: Teen Pregnancy:* http://youtu.be/Vjdd41VbNvk

Exercise 6-27: *True or false*
Stephanie knows that teenagers, girls and boys alike, typically engage in sexual activity to express emotions related to love.

    A. True

    B. False

Exercise 6-28: *Select all that apply*
Which of the following statements regarding children born to teenage mothers are correct?

    ❑ Children born to teenage mothers are more likely to have developmental delays.

    ❑ Children born to teenage mothers are likely to receive proper nutrition, health care, and cognitive and social stimulation.

    ❑ Children born to teenage mothers are on an equal footing with other children in potential for academic achievement.

    ❑ Children born to teenage mothers are at increased risk for abuse and neglect.

Exercise 6-29: *True or false*
Boys born to teenage mothers are no more likely to be incarcerated later in life than their counterparts.

    A. True

    B. False

Exercise 6-30: *True or false*
Girls born to teenage mothers are more likely to become teenage mothers themselves.

    A. True

    B. False

Exercise 6-31: *Multiple-choice question*
_____ of teen pregnancies are unplanned

    A. 50%

    B. 74%

    C. 82%

    D. 90%

Answers to this chapter begin on page 154.

Stephanie decides to put into place a comprehensive teenage pregnancy prevention program. She wants to make sure that she is approaching the problem from primary, secondary, and tertiary prevention levels.

Exercise 6-32: *Fill-in*

What can the nurse do to address the problem of teenage pregnancy at the primary prevention level?

Exercise 6-33: *Fill-in*

What can the nurse do to address the problem of teenage pregnancy at the secondary prevention level?

_____

_____

_____

_____

Exercise 6-34: *Multiple-choice question*

Which of the following would be considered secondary prevention for teen pregnancy?

     A. Sex education program

     B. Pregnancy resolution services

     C. Parenting skills program

     D. Access to contraceptives

Stephanie organizes a workshop for the parents, teachers, and staff at the school. As part of the session, she plans to provide a handout that gives an overview of the current statistics related to teenage pregnancy.

 eResource 6-10: CDC's Guide: *Teen Pregnancy: Improving the Lives of Young People and Strengthening Communities by Reducing Teen Pregnancy*: http://goo.gl/iNDF6

Stephanie prepares for her presentation by listening to a presentation that provides information regarding the social impact of teenage pregnancy.

 eResource 6-11: To highlight the impact of poverty and pregnancy, Stephanie plays a brief excerpt from Radio Health Journal's podcast, The Pregnant Poor: [Pathway: http://goo.gl/ALjtd → scroll down and locate "The Pregnant Poor"] (air date: January 6, 2012)

Stephanie considers Lewin's Change Theory in her preparations. She knows that providing this information is essential in encouraging the change for which she is hoping.

Answers to this chapter begin on page 154.

Figure 6-6: Lewin's Change Theory

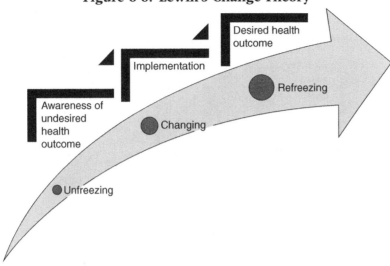

Source: Adapted from Lewin (1951).

Exercise 6-35: *Fill-in*

Describe activities that Stephanie will likely engage in at each stage of the change process.

Table 6-1

Stage	Activities
Unfreezing	
Changing	
Refreezing	

Stephanie knows that in order to make a change in teenage pregnancy, teens must have knowledge of sexual health, HIV infection, other sexually transmitted diseases (STDs), and pregnancy (including methods of prevention). But it is important that the adults in the community do their part too. So Stephanie's goals include a variety of measures that include heightened awareness by the parents, teachers, and staff at the school. To provide visual impact regarding the prevalence of teenage pregnancy among African Americans and Hispanics, Stephanie shows the attendees a graph.

Answers to this chapter begin on page 154.

Figure 6-7: Birth Rates Among U.S. Females Aged 15–19 Years, by Race/Ethnicity, 2005–2009

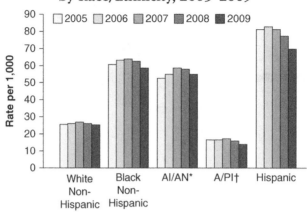

* American Indian/Alaska Native
† Asian American/Pacific Islander

Source: CDC, National Center for Health Statistics.

 eResource 6-12: To get the discussion going, she shows a video, *Answers for Preventing Teen Pregnancy*: http://youtu.be/_nqY1HF4JgQ

After watching the video, Stephanie facilitates a lively discussion regarding what can be done to prevent teen pregnancies in the community.

Unfolding Case Study #3 ▨ Mental Health in the Community

Olivia Patterson is a nurse working in the local public health department. As part of her caseload, she visits individuals living in the community who have mental health issues. Olivia knows that the mentally ill are a vulnerable population and are at greater risk for poor health outcomes.

Exercise 6-36: *Multiple-choice question*
Which of the following statements about the mentally ill is true?

    A. Mental illness is primarily an age-related manifestation.

    B. The mentally ill are at no greater risk of substance abuse than other groups.

    C. The mentally ill are at high risk of suicide.

    D. One third of people in nursing homes have a mental illness.

Answers to this chapter begin on page 154.

Exercise 6-37: *Fill-in*

Factors that contribute to mental illness include:

_____

_____

_____

_____

Sammy is a young man living in a group home who has been diagnosed as having schizophrenia. Olivia makes a home visit to see how Sammy is doing and also to assess his response to his medication regimen. As part of the comprehensive community base support services, Olivia works with a team that includes a physician and social services. Olivia realizes that just like her other patients, Sammy has basic needs.

Exercise 6-38: *Fill-in*

The goal of the team caring for Sammy is to keep him living in the community with an optimal quality of life. This includes:

_____

_____

_____

_____

Olivia is also interested in the mental health of the community she serves. She knows that mental illness affects a growing number of people and according to the World Health Organization, "accounts for more disability in developed countries than any other group of illnesses, including cancer and heart disease" (CDC, September 2, 2011, p. 1). She collaborates with her colleagues to put into place a program to address mental illness in the community because mental illness is a growing public health problem (Centers for Disease Control and Prevention., 2011d).

Exercise 6-39: *Fill-in*

List the interventions that Olivia and her colleagues can implement to address mental illness in the community from primary, secondary, and tertiary levels of prevention.

Table 6-2

Level	Interventions
Primary prevention	
Secondary prevention	
Tertiary prevention	

Olivia is conducting a depression screening within a community. During the screening, she assesses Hector Gallo, a 36-year-old man who tells her that he has been divorced for 6 months. His two children, aged 13 and 15, are now living with their mother. The children refuse to talk to or see him. He reports that he has lost

Answers to this chapter begin on page 154.

20 pounds since the divorce and says he lacks motivation to get out of the house to do anything besides going to work. He also reports that he has difficulty falling asleep at night. He says he does not want to be labeled as "weird" for seeing a psychiatrist for mental health concerns.

Exercise 6-40: *Fill-in*

What factors are adversely affecting the mental health of this client?

_____

_____

_____

_____

Exercise 6-41: *Fill-in*

What interventions are warranted for Mr. Gallo?

_____

_____

_____

_____

Unfolding Case Study #4 ▦ Substance Abuse

Melanie is a nurse practitioner working in a community-based clinic. She has a follow-up visit with Peter, a 24-year-old who broke his ankle while drinking at a party several weeks ago. Peter's ankle is healing as expected without complications. Peter tells Melanie that he has been wondering if his drinking is "Okay." He says he has never been arrested for driving intoxicated, nor has he experienced any health or relationship problems. Melanie asks him some additional questions. Peter tells her that he called in sick to work one time and drove intoxicated several times.

Exercise 6-42: *Fill-in*

What questions should Melanie ask Peter?

_____

_____

_____

_____

 eResource 6-13: Melanie consults an Alcohol Abuse Screening Test (http://goo.gl/qT9Id) and uses the tool to guide additional follow-up questions.

Answers to this chapter begin on page 154.

Exercise 6-43: *Multiple-choice question*

Melanie responds to Peter that he may have a drinking problem because:

     A. "You are drinking more than two drinks per occasion."

     B. "You seem to have the inability to stop drinking despite negative consequences."

     C. "You have experienced drinking that causes you to pass out or experience a blackout."

     D. "You are drinking too much and too often and are using poor judgment with negative consequences."

 eResource 6-14: Melanie shows Peter a web-based self-assessment tool from the Mayo Clinic: http://goo.gl/HDYrl

Exercise 6-44: *Multiple-choice question*

What level of prevention is appropriate when working with this client at the clinic?

     A. Primary

     B. Secondary

     C. Tertiary

     D. Rehabilitation

Exercise 6-45: *Fill-in*

What are some examples of interventions that Melanie should make?

_____

_____

_____

_____

_____

Answers to this chapter begin on page 154.

Answers

Exercise 6-1: *Fill-in*

What does it mean to be vulnerable? Provide an example of a vulnerable patient.

To be vulnerable means to be susceptible to negative events and little or no control over the effects of these events. It can be manifested by an interaction of internal and external factors. Example: Person with COPD who lives in area with severe air pollution.

Exercise 6-2: *Fill-in*

Define vulnerable populations.

As it relates to health, to be vulnerable is to be at greater risk for illness or disability than others are. Vulnerable populations have an increased risk for developing adverse health outcomes. Vulnerable populations have less control over their health than the general population. There is usually an interaction among poverty, housing, financial and social resources, environment, access to care, and family physical and emotional history.

Exercise 6-3: *Fill-in*

Which populations are considered vulnerable populations?

Vulnerable populations include:

- **the economically disadvantaged**
- **racial and ethnic minorities**
- **the uninsured**
- **low-income children**
- **the elderly**
- **the homeless**
- **those with HIV**
- **those with other chronic health conditions**
- **severe mental illness**
- **survivors of violence**
- **pregnant adolescents**
- **immigrants**
- **substance abusers**
- **prisoners/ex-convicts**
- **individuals who have limited access to or encounter barriers to health care service**

Exercise 6-4: *Select all that apply*

Vulnerable populations frequently have less control over their health due to:

☒ **Socioeconomic factors**

☒ **Income**

☒ **Education**

☒ **Access issues**

☒ **Health beliefs**

☒ **Disenfranchisement**

Exercise 6-5: *Fill-in*

What factors contribute to vulnerability?

- **Poverty**
- **Livelihood**
- **Cultural beliefs**
- **Equity**
- **Gender**
- **Weaker social groups**
- **Financial circumstances**
- **Place of residence**
- **Health**
- **Age**
- **Functional or developmental status**
- **Ability to communicate effectively**
- **Race**
- **Ethnicity**

Exercise 6-6: *Fill-in*

What are the broader public health implications associated with the health of vulnerable populations?

Core function of assurance is "providing essential personal health services for those who would otherwise not receive them" (HealthyPeople.gov, 2012). But the health (or lack of health) of these individuals can have wider societal impact. For example, farmworkers come in contact with the nation's food supply and therefore could impact the health of others. In addition, pregnant adolescents who do not get good prenatal care risk having premature babies, babies with health problems, and so forth, which has implications for future generations. In another example, violence has a far-reaching impact on the community.

Exercise 6-7: *Multiple-choice question*

An example of an individual from a vulnerable population is:

A. **Person with asthma who lives next to a factory that manufactures tires—YES, this indicates environmental pollution that can affect health.**

B. Person with COPD who lives next to a pharmacy—NO, this person has access.

C. Person with a cold who is not taking antibiotics—NO, this person is making a choice.

D. Person with a 3-cm area of erythema 24 hours after a PPD test—NO, it must be 5 cm to be significant.

Exercise 6-8: *Multiple-choice question*

Which of the following best reflects the definition of a vulnerable population?

A. The homeless population in a large city—NO, this person is at risk but does not define all vulnerable individuals.

B. Groups that are susceptible to certain communicable diseases—NO, this group is at risk, but does not define all vulnerable individuals.

C. **Groups that have an increased risk to develop adverse health outcome—YES**

D. Groups that live in low-income housing—NO, this group is at risk but does not define all vulnerable individuals.

Exercise 6-9: *Multiple-choice question*
All of the following are examples of a vulnerable population except:
A. Severely mentally ill—NO, this makes a person vulnerable.
B. Migrant workers—NO, this makes a person vulnerable.
C. Impoverished population—NO, this makes a person vulnerable.
D. Nursing students—YES, learners are not vulnerable.

Exercise 6-10: *Fill-in*
Define poverty:

Poverty is defined as having an insufficient income to meet basic living expenses for food, shelter, clothing, transportation, and health care.

Exercise 6-11: *Fill-in*
What is the federal poverty level? How is it determined?

In January of each year, the federal government announces an official income level for poverty called the Federal Poverty Income Guidelines. This is frequently referred to as the "Federal Poverty Level." Benefit levels of low-income assistance programs are based on these poverty guidelines. It is important to note that a pregnant woman counts as two for the purpose of calculating Federal Poverty Income Guidelines.

Exercise 6-12: *Multiple-choice question*
_____ is a concept that implies that some people are worthy to have a roof over their heads and others not.
A. Maleficence—NO, this is an ethical dilemma.
B. Distributive justice—YES
C. Creative justice—NO, this is nondiscriminating.
D. Fair and Equal Division of Resource Act—NO, this is nondiscriminating.

Exercise 6-13: *Fill-in*
What is resiliency?

Resiliency is a phenomenon associated with an individual's ability to resist the impact of factors that contribute to poor health outcomes. Some members of a vulnerable population don't "succumb" to poor health outcomes. This is a very interesting phenomenon that has been a focus of study to help us understand why some individuals are more resistant to poor health outcomes than their counterparts.

Exercise 6-14: *Fill-in*

What is the Latino Paradox?

 eResource 6-15: To learn more about the Latino Paradox, view: http://goo.gl/icS4k

The Latino Paradox refers to the finding that Latinos in the United States have overall mortality rates and infant mortality rates, two standard measures of a population's health, approaching and sometimes lower than that of Whites. This is puzzling to public health experts, given the link between disadvantage and high disease and mortality rates (Chung, 2006).

Exercise 6-15: *Fill-in*

What are the overarching goals of Healthy People 2020?

The overarching goals of Healthy People 2020 are:

1. **Attain high-quality, longer lives free of preventable disease, disability, injury, and premature death.**
2. **Achieve health equity, eliminate disparities, and improve the health of all groups.**
3. **Create social and physical environments that promote good health for all.**
4. **Promote quality of life, healthy development, and healthy behaviors across all life stages (HealthyPeople.gov, 2012).**

Exercise 6-16: *Fill-in*

How does poverty influence vulnerability?

The poor tend to be

- **Marginalized and disenfranchised**
- **Politically invisible**
- **Don't vote**
- **Seldom organized**
- **Don't own property**
- **Of low social status**
- **Disproportionately minorities**
- **Disproportionately female—"feminization of poverty"**
- **A poor inner-city population where middle class does not travel**
- **Rates of poverty are highest in women of color and lowest among White males**
- **Age (very young and very elderly); children are disproportionately represented**
- **Poor health status—or multiple chronic illnesses**

Figure 6-8: Health Status Related to Income

(The lower the income, the greater the incidence of chronic health problems)

	Heart disease	Coronary heart disease	Heart attack	Stroke	Cancer, all	Arthritis	Diabetes
All	11.5	6.4	3.1	2.6	8.2	21.6	8.7
Poor	14.7	9.1	4.7	4.7	6.4	25.1	12.1
Near poor	13.1	8.1	4.2	4.0	7.7	23.5	11.0
Nonpoor	10.7	5.6	2.6	2.0	8.6	20.6	7.7

Notes: Family income expressed as a percent of the poverty threshold. Reported and imputed income levels were grouped into three categories: poor (<100% of the poverty threshold), near poor (100% to <200% of the poverty threshold), and nonpoor (200% of the poverty threshold or greater).

Exercise 6-17: *Multiple-choice question*

Poverty is defined as:

A. **Having insufficient financial resources to meet basic living expenses for food, clothing, shelter, transportation, and health care—YES**

B. A family of four with income less than $32,000—NO, this does not tell the whole picture.

C. A homeless man that goes to the St. John's Hospice daily for lunch—NO, this does not tell the whole picture.

D. Having insufficient financial resources to meet their mortgage payments on a monthly basis—NO, this does not tell the whole picture because money is needed for food also.

Exercise 6-18: *Fill-in*

What factors make Billy vulnerable?

- **Billy is a child living in poverty**
- **He is a minority**
- **Risky neighborhood—recruited by gangs**
- **Poor academic performance at risk for failure**
- **Lack of sleep**
- **Poor nutrition**

Exercise 6-19: *Fill-in*

What are the issues/concerns for Billy?

- **Socioeconomic factors adversely affect health**
- **Poor health behaviors—lack of sleep, nutrition**
- **Stress**
- **At risk for failing out of high school**

Exercise 6-20: *Fill-in*

Identify interventions for Billy at primary, secondary, and tertiary levels for one of the issues/concerns identified in the previous exercise.

Ideally the following interventions would be possible; however, the situation that Billy is in is much more complex and warrants a community/family approach to support healthy behaviors and positive health outcomes.

1. **Primary prevention:**
   a. **Stress reduction: Living wage for Billy's father, so Billy does not have to work and can focus upon his studies**
   b. **Healthy lifestyle: sufficient sleep, good nutrition, physical activity**
2. **Secondary prevention: School remediation; academic tutoring to support learning and completing assignments**
3. **Tertiary prevention: None warranted at this point as Billy does not yet present with disease/illness/negative health outcomes**

Exercise 6-21: *Fill-in*

What factors make the Elkins' family vulnerable?

- **Low socioeconomic status**
- **Lack of education/marketable skills**
- **Lack of access to affordable healthy food**
- **Multiple chronic health problems**
- **Deferred health care**

Exercise 6-22: *Fill-in*

What are the issues/concerns for the Elkins' family?

1. **Inadequate financial resources**
2. **Declining health, chronic health problems, and inability to effectively manage illnesses**
3. **History of stroke twice (Clint)**
4. **Stress**

Exercise 6-23: *Fill-in*

Identify interventions for the Elkins' family at the primary, secondary, and tertiary levels for one of the issues/concerns identified in the previous exercise.

The situation experienced by the Elkins' family is also very complex and warrants a community/family approach to support healthy behaviors and positive health outcomes.

1. Primary prevention:

    a. Stress reduction: a key component of this would be not to have to worry about finances, but also it is about caregiver burden (consideration of this for both Sheryl [caregiving for Ester and Yvonne as well as her autistic son] and Ester [caregiving for her husband Clint])

    b. Healthy lifestyle: good nutrition, physical activity, adequate rest

    c. Improved financial status—directly linked to health status

2. Secondary prevention: Diabetes education; diabetic diet and self-care; minimizing

3. Tertiary prevention: Rehabilitation of Clint following second stroke; therapies to reduce/prevent risk for another stroke

Exercise 6-24: *Multiple-choice question*

Stephanie is working with teens in a high school life skills class. They are discussing attitudes and feelings about smoking; the nurse uses role playing as a teaching tool. This is an example of which of the following domains of learning?

A. Cognitive—NO, this is the thinking domain.

B. Psychomotor—NO, this is the "doing" domain.

C. Affective—YES, this is the feeling domain.

D. Teaching—NO

Exercise 6-25: *Fill-in*

Teen pregnancy is a concern because:

Teenage mothers

- **Are less likely to have prenatal care**
- **Have poorer eating habits**
- **More likely to smoke, drink alcohol, or take drugs during pregnancy**
- **Less likely to gain adequate weight during their pregnancy, leading to low birth weight**
- **Teens are children themselves, with bodies not yet fully developed**

Babies of teenage moms are more likely to have low birth weight, which is linked to

- **Increased infant mortality**
- **Disorders such as bleeding in the brain, respiratory distress syndrome, and intestinal problems because organs are not fully developed**

Exercise 6-26: *Fill-in*

Factors that contribute to teenage pregnancy include:

- <u>**Being sexually active**</u>
- <u>**Lack of access to or poor use of contraception**</u>
- <u>**Living in poverty**</u>
- <u>**Having parents with low levels of education**</u>
- <u>**Poor performance in school**</u>
- <u>**Growing up in a single-parent family**</u>
- <u>**The influence of an older sibling**</u>
- <u>**The perception that peers are sexually active**</u>
- <u>**Early pubertal development**</u>
- <u>**Sexual abuse**</u>
- <u>**Alcohol and drug use**</u>
- <u>**Hormonal changes and sexual awareness**</u>
- <u>**Peer pressure**</u>
- <u>**Pervasive sexual messages in the media**</u>
- <u>**Involuntary sexual activity**</u>
- <u>**Inaccuracy or lack of knowledge regarding sex and contraception**</u>
- <u>**Misuse or nonuse of contraception**</u>
- <u>**Difficulty of access to birth control**</u>
- <u>**Destigmatization of illegitimacy**</u>
- <u>**Efforts at independence**</u>
- <u>**Need to feel special, loved, and wanted**</u>
- <u>**Lack of future orientation and maturity**</u>

Exercise 6-27: *True or false*

Stephanie knows that teenagers, girls and boys alike, typically engage in sexual activity to express emotions related to love.

A. True
B. **False**

Exhibit 6-2: Answer Details

Teenage girls typically engage in sexual activity to express emotions and closeness related to love, while the boys engage in sex for pleasure rather than for emotional closeness.

Exercise 6-28: *Select all that apply*

Which of the following statements regarding children born to teenage mothers are correct?

☒ **Children born to teenage mothers are more likely to have developmental delays.**

❑ Children born to teenage mothers are likely to receive proper nutrition, health care, and cognitive and social stimulation.

❑ Children born to teenage mothers are on equal footing with other children in potential for academic achievement.

☒ **Children born to teenage mothers are at increased risk for abuse and neglect.**

Exercise 6-29: *True or false*

Boys born to teenage mothers are no more likely to be incarcerated later in life than their counterparts.

A. True

B. False—YES, boys born to teenage mothers are 13% more likely to be incarcerated later in life (Guttmacher Institute, 2012).

Exercise 6-30: *True or false*

Girls born to teenage mothers are more likely to become teenage mothers themselves.

A. True—YES, girls born to teenage mothers are 22% more likely to become teenage mothers themselves (Guttmacher Institute, 2012).

B. False

Exercise 6-31: *Multiple-choice question*

_____ of teen pregnancies are unplanned

A. 50%

B. 74%

C. 82%

D. 90%

Exercise 6-32: *Fill-in*

What can the nurse do to address the problem of teenage pregnancy at the primary prevention level?

<u>Primary prevention</u>

- **<u>Delay or stop participation in sexual activity</u>**
- **<u>Provide access to contraceptives</u>**
- **<u>Strengthen future life goals</u>**

- **Education!! Comprehensive sex education is most effective**
- **Contraceptive services**
- **Life options or youth development programs**

Exercise 6-33: *Fill-in*

What can the nurse do to address the problem of teenage pregnancy at the secondary prevention level?

- **Early detection**
- **Counseling and support**
- **Shelter/housing services**
- **Pregnancy resolution services**
  - **Abortion**
  - **Adoption**
- **Prenatal health care/prenatal programs**
- **Childbirth education**
- **Special needs of adolescents—developmental, physical, educational**
- **Postpartum and newborn care**
- **Parenting classes**
- **Support systems and nurse home visits**
- **Health status of new mom**
- **Role adjustment**
- **Health status of newborn**
- **Depression screening**
- **General health teaching**
- **Adolescent and young adult father care and engagement**

Exercise 6-34: *Multiple-choice question*

Which of the following would be considered secondary prevention for teen pregnancy?

A. Sex education program—NO, this is primary.
B. Pregnancy resolution services—YES
C. Parenting skills program—NO, this is tertiary.
D. Access to contraceptives—NO, this is primary.

Exercise 6-35: *Fill-in*

Describe activities that Stephanie will likely engage in at each stage of the change process.

Table 6-3

Stage	Activities
Unfreezing	**Providing information regarding** • **pregnancy statistics (national, state, regional, and district)** • **untoward outcomes of teen pregnancy** • **success stories (best practices, programs that work)**
Changing	**Organize prevention activities** • **Education campaign** • **Comprehensive sex education curricula or youth development programs** • **Access to information regarding birth control**
Refreezing	**Continue funding and support to sustain programs** **Evaluate effectiveness to determine if new approaches are warranted**

Exercise 6-36: *Multiple-choice question*

Which of the following statements about the mentally ill is true?

A. Mental illness is primarily an age-related manifestation—NO, it can strike at any age.

B. The mentally ill are at no greater risk of substance abuse than other groups—NO, they are at increased risk.

C. The mentally ill are at high risk of suicide—YES

D. One third of people in nursing homes have a mental illness—NO, this is not true.

Exercise 6-37: *Fill-in*

Factors that contribute to mental illness include:

- **Individual coping abilities (poor coping)**
- **Stressful life events (exposure to violence)**
- **Social events (recent divorce, bereavement, other losses)**
- **Chronic health problems**
- **Stigma associated with seeking mental health services**

Exercise 6-38: *Fill-in*

The goal of the team caring for Sammy is to keep him living in the community with an optimal quality of life. This includes:

To help Sammy maintain a level of function that allows him to live in the community, the team strives to make sure that he has:

- **A safe living environment**
- **Basic life necessities**

- **Access to medication and health care**
- **Support from family/caregivers**
- **Emotional/psychosocial needs are met**
- **A sense that life is meaningful**

Exercise 6-39: *Fill-in*

List the interventions that Olivia and her colleagues can implement to address mental illness in the community from primary, secondary, and tertiary levels of prevention.

Table 6-4

Level	Interventions
Primary prevention	**Educate populations regarding mental health issues**
	Teach stress reduction techniques
	Provide parenting classes
	Provide bereavement support
	Promote protective factors (coping) and risk factor reduction
	Advocate for rights of mentally ill
Secondary prevention	**Screen to detect mental health disorders (case finding and referrals)**
	Work directly with individuals, families, and groups
	Conduct crisis intervention
	Perform medication monitoring
	Provide mental health interventions
Tertiary prevention	**Referrals to professionals and support groups**
	Identify behavioral, environmental, and biological triggers that may lead to relapse
	Assist in planning to minimize sources of stress
	Education regarding medication side effects, interactions
	Advocate for rehab and recovery services

Exercise 6-40: *Fill-in*

What factors are adversely affecting the mental health of this client?

- **Recent divorce**
- **Children not speaking to or interacting with him**
- **Perceived stigma associated with seeking mental health services**
- **Social isolation**

Exercise 6-41: *Fill-in*

What interventions are warranted for Mr. Gallo?

- **Reassurance that seeking help will not "label" him; provide information regarding typical responses to life events such as divorce**
- **Referral to counseling**
- **Referral to support group for divorced people**
- **Encourage Mr. Gallo to speak to his primary health care provider regarding his concerns**
- **Provide patient teaching material**

Exercise 6-42: *Fill-in*

What questions should Melanie ask Peter?

- **How often do you consume alcohol?**
- **How much do you drink at a time?**
- **Has your frequency increased or decreased over the past month?**
- **Have you missed classes or work because of the use of alcohol?**
- **Have you increased the amount of alcohol that you consume to obtain the effects that you used to have after a smaller amount of alcohol?**

Exercise 6-43: *Multiple-choice question*

Melanie responds to Peter that he may have a drinking problem because:

A. "You are drinking more than two drinks per occasion."—NO, this does not define alcoholism.

B. "You seem to have the inability to stop drinking despite negative consequences."—NO, this does not define alcoholism.

C. "You have experienced drinking that causes you to pass out or experience a blackout."—NO, this does not define alcoholism.

D. "You are drinking too much and too often and are using poor judgment with negative consequences."—YES, it is affecting functioning.

Exhibit 6-3: Answer Details

Peter reports drinking and driving. This fits the abuse category as "recurrent substance use in hazardous situations." This reflects poor judgment. In addition, his recent injury may be further evidence that he has a drinking problem that contributed to the injury.

Exercise 6-44: *Multiple-choice question*

What level of prevention is appropriate when working with this client at the clinic?

A. Primary—NO, it is too late for primary.

B. Secondary—YES

C. Tertiary—NO, there are no complications.

D. Rehabilitation—NO

Exercise 6-45: *Fill-in*

What are some examples of interventions that Melanie should make?

- **Assess habits and history related to excessive alcohol consumption and use**

- **In a nonjudgmental way, educate the client about the effects of alcohol, risks of drinking and driving, and the importance of preventing another motor vehicle crash**

- **Explore readiness and motivation to change his behavior**

- **Explore alternative activities and college programs for recreation**

- **If he chooses to make behavior changes, refer the client to a support group and/or counselor if necessary**

- **If he chooses not to make immediate changes, encourage him to follow up with another appointment and think about a decision that will promote health**

7

Health Promotion

Unfolding Case Study #1 ▦ Dominique Jones— Kindergarten Round-Up

Marilee Dibbler is a nurse practitioner (NP) working in a large urban school district in Portland, Oregon. On an annual basis, she coordinates "Kindergarten Round-Up" programs with the local health department to help facilitate the process of ensuring that all children are prepared to enter school in the fall. As part of this endeavor, she makes sure that parents receive information and are linked to available resources well in advance.

 eResource 7-1: Some of the resources Marilee makes available include:
- The ABCs of Kindergarten: http://goo.gl/Tw0df
- Immunization requirements: http://goo.gl/AmCyh

Dominique Jones, a 4½-year-old only child, is taken by her mother, Tonya, to the Kindergarten Round-Up Immunization Clinic held at Kroder Elementary School for immunizations in preparation for entering kindergarten. Dominique has not been to the doctor since her 3-year-old checkup so doesn't really remember much about that visit. Tonya tries to prepare Dominique for the visit by telling her what to expect. Dominique lives with her mother and two older brothers in an older rented duplex in the north side of the city.

Exercise 7-1: *Select all that apply*
Which of the components of a typical well-child exam should Dominique expect?
- ❏ Height
- ❏ Head circumference
- ❏ Weight
- ❏ Blood pressure
- ❏ Sexually transmitted infection (STI) screening
- ❏ Dyslipidemia screening
- ❏ Development

Answers to this chapter begin on page 181.

❏ Body mass index (BMI)

❏ Vision test

❏ Hearing test

❏ Tuberculosis test

e **eResource 7-2:** To learn more about Recommendations for Preventive Pediatric Health Care from the American Academy of Pediatrics and Bright Futures, go to: http://goo.gl/Al6JQ

After the NP conducts the routine physical assessment, she reviews Dominique's immunization record.

Exercise 7-2: *Select all that apply*

What are the routine immunizations that should be administered to Dominique?

❏ DTaP

❏ IPV

❏ HepB

❏ MMR

❏ PVC

❏ Varicella

Exercise 7-3: *Fill-in*

Marilee knows that in addition to performing a physical assessment, it is also important for the nurse to assess for:

_____

_____

_____

_____

Tonya is eager to help Dominique prepare for school. She is concerned because Dominique has not had the opportunity to attend preschool and so may have difficulty adjusting. "I worry since she has been home with me and may have problems being apart from me." Marilee tells Tonya that there are things that she can do over the next several months to help Dominique prepare for school.

Exercise 7-4: *Multiple-choice question*

Marilee remembers Erikson's Stages of Psychosocial Development and realizes that Dominique is likely at which of the following stages:

A. Initiative versus guilt

B. Trust versus mistrust

C. Industry versus inferiority

D. Autonomy versus shame and doubt

Answers to this chapter begin on page 181.

Exercise 7-5: *Multiple-choice question*

Marilee also realizes that at this time, Dominique is learning to:

 A. Develop a sense of trust when caregivers provide reliability, care, and affection

 B. Develop a sense of personal control over physical skills and a sense of independence

 C. Develop the ability to try new things and learn how to handle failure

 D. Develop a sense of pride in accomplishments and abilities

 E. Develop a sense of self and personal identity

 F. Form intimate, loving relationships with other people

 eResource 7-3: Marilee provides Tonya with several parenting resources:

 ▪ *Ready, Set, Connect to Kindergarten*: A parent guide with activities to help Dominique prepare for school: http://goo.gl/jRS78

 ▪ The ABCs of Kindergarten: http://goo.gl/Tw0df

 ▪ PBS's *The Whole Child*: http://goo.gl/DnXWp

Exercise 7-6: *Multiple-choice question*

By providing Tonya these materials, Marilee is engaging in which of the following:

 A. Proactive education

 B. Anticipatory guidance

 C. Primary prevention

 D. Secondary prevention

Exercise 7-7: *Multiple-choice question*

Marilee also knows that the leading cause of death for children Dominique's age is:

 A. Infectious disease

 B. Unintentional injury

 C. Motor vehicle accidents

 D. Congenital anomalies

Exercise 7-8: *Multiple-choice question*

In comparison with other high-income countries, the death rate for children under the age of 14 in the United States is ranked:

 A. Among the lowest

 B. Third

 C. Fifth

 D. Sixth

Marilee knows that in addition to anticipatory guidance, prevention of injuries requires environmental modification and safety education.

Answers to this chapter begin on page 181.

Exercise 7-9: *Fill-in*
What primary prevention measures can Tonya put into place to protect Dominique?

_____

_____

_____

_____

_____

_____

 eResource 7-4: Marilee gives some additional materials to Tonya that supplement the anticipatory guidance provided: http://goo.gl/MSi1Y

Tonya has heard a lot in the news about the upcoming flu season and predictions that this year's flu season will be particularly harsh. Tonya asks the nurse, "Dominique has never received the flu shot. Should she also get the flu shot today?"

Exercise 7-10: *Multiple-choice question*
What would the correct response to Tonya be?
    A. "Dominique doesn't need the flu shot; she is still protected by the natural immunity from breast feeding."
    B. "Dominique is young and healthy; if all of her other immunizations are up to date, she does not need the flu shot."
    C. "Dominique should receive the flu shot today and every year to protect her from the influenza virus."
    D. "Dominique should receive the flu shot today and another dose in 4 weeks."

Exercise 7-11: *Multiple-choice question*
Before the nurse gives Dominique the flu shot, which of the following questions should she ask Tonya?
    A. "Have you noticed any unusual behavior in Dominique lately?"
    B. "Did Dominique vomit today?"
    C. "When was the last time Dominique ate?"
    D. "Is Dominique allergic to eggs?"

Tonya says to the nurse, "I know everyone says that you should get the flu shot but it seems to me that people still get the flu. The shot doesn't keep you from getting the flu."

Answers to this chapter begin on page 181.

Exercise 7-12: *Multiple-choice question*

What would be the best response for the nurse to give?

    A. "People who get the flu shot are protected from the flu virus immediately."

    B. "It takes 4 weeks (1 month) for the flu vaccination to take full effect, so if you are exposed to the flu during that time, you might get the flu."

    C. "Some illnesses have flulike symptoms, so people may mistakenly think that they have caught the flu even after getting the flu shot."

    D. "Getting the flu shot can lessen the severity of illness."

    E. B and C

    F. C and D

    G. A, C, and D

Marilee spends time answering all of Tonya's questions regarding the flu vaccine and what to expect after Dominique receives the flu shot.

 eResource 7-5: Marilee provides Tonya with additional educational materials:

    ■ A brochure entitled *The Flu: A Guide for Parent*s, which gives an overview of measures to take to reduce risk: http://goo.gl/M9hTn

    ■ *Teaching Children About the Flu:* http://goo.gl/HaHhN

    ■ *Cover Your Cough*, a visual aid to help reduce transmission: http://goo.gl/n8E56

Tonya tells Marilee that she is pregnant and asks, "Is it safe for me to get the flu shot?"

Exercise 7-13: *True or false*

Is the influenza vaccination safe for pregnant women?

    A. True

    B. False

Exercise 7-14: *Multiple-choice question*

Tonya still has questions about the flu shot and how this can affect her pregnancy. Which of the following statements made by Marilee is most accurate?

    A. "The changes that occur in your body when you are pregnant build immunity against illness, so you don't need the flu shot."

    B. "While pregnant women are at no greater risk from influenza as the general public, you should still get the vaccination."

    C. "Pregnant women with influenza are at no greater risk for premature labor than their counterparts."

    D. "Getting the influenza vaccine will protect your unborn baby and protect the baby after birth."

    E. "Since you are pregnant, it is best that you get the nasal spray flu vaccine."

Answers to this chapter begin on page 181.

eResource 7-6: Marilee provides additional patient education materials to Tonya:
- *Protect Yourself, Protect Your Baby*: http://youtu.be/3J5ijqtmkPk
- *Pregnant Women Need the Flu Shot*: http://goo.gl/cc75g

Unfolding Case Study #2 ▨ School Health Program

Warren West is a school nurse working in a suburban elementary school near Boston, Massachusetts. As the school nurse, Warren is responsible for the oversight of the provision of school health services and health promotion education at the school. These activities are often either community-based, population-focused, or both.

Exercise 7-15: *Fill-in*
The National Association of School Nurses identifies seven core roles of the school nurse. List the core roles and provide a specific example of an activity for each.

1. _____

2. _____

3. _____

4. _____

5. _____

6. _____

7. _____

In his role as the school nurse, Warren provides primary, secondary, and tertiary care to the students and staff of the school.

Exercise 7-16: *Fill-in*
Identify which of the following is primary (P), secondary (S), or tertiary (T) care.

_____ Health services for students with special needs

_____ Health education

_____ Healthful school environment

_____ Physical education

_____ Counseling, psychological, and social services

_____ Site health promotion for faculty and staff

_____ Primary care

_____ Case management

Answers to this chapter begin on page 181.

_____ Administration of medications

_____ Managing minor complaints, scrapes, headache, etc.

_____ Immunizations status

_____ Health screening

Exercise 7-17: *Multiple-choice question*

An example of tertiary prevention that Warren provides would be:

    A. Conducting screening tests or arranging for screening by others

    B. Providing first aid for a fall injury

    C. Providing safety education

    D. Providing for special equipment needs

Warren has been asked by the principal to organize the school's self-study to evaluate the health programs offered at the school. Warren is aware that the CDC has developed a guide to help schools conduct this comprehensive self-assessment and plans to review this prior to moving forward (Centers for Disease Control and Prevention Division of Adolescent and School Health, 2005).

 eResource 7-7: Warren locates and reviews the CDC School Health Index (SHI): A Self-Assessment and Planning Guide: http://goo.gl/vytYM

Using the guide as a reference, Warren decides to call a meeting, inviting all the key stakeholders to attend.

Exercise 7-18: *Fill-in*

Who are the key stakeholders that Warren should invite to this meeting?

_____

_____

_____

 eResource 7-8: Prior to this meeting, Warren reviews another resource provided by the CDC, Steps for Conducting a SHI Training: http://goo.gl/fGKNR

Warren also knows that in order to move forward on a school self-assessment, he needs to build consensus among the key stakeholders.

Exercise 7-19: *Multiple-choice question*

Consensus is:

    A. A unanimous vote

    B. A majority vote

    C. Everyone 100% satisfied

    D. A solution that all members can support

At the meeting, Warren introduces his proposal to do a School Health Index. He tells the audience that there are eight components of a coordinated school health program and describes the services that are currently being offered at the school.

Figure 7-1: Components of Coordinated School Health Program

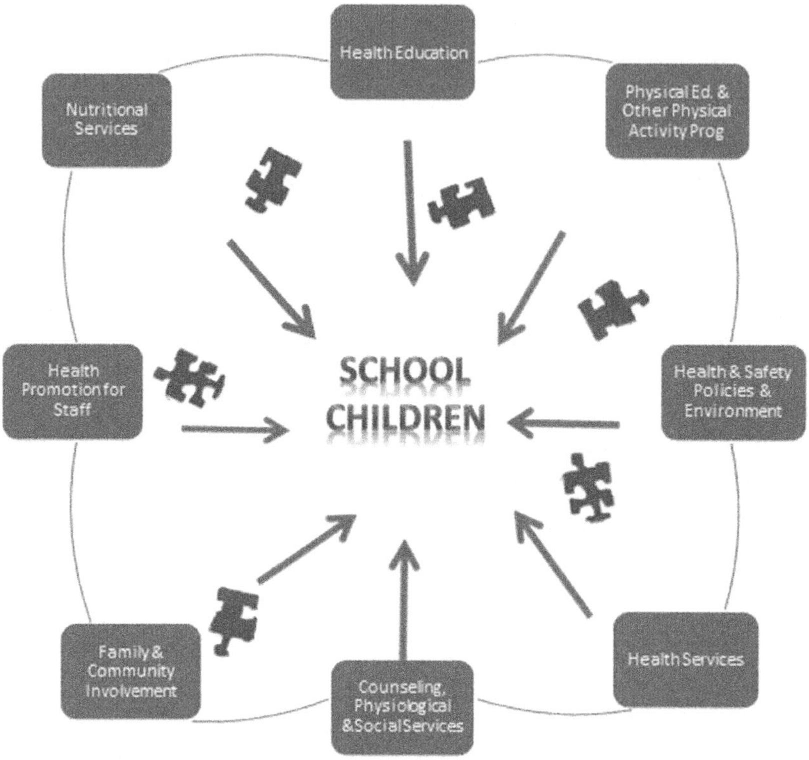

Source: Adapted from CDC Division of Adolescent and School Health (2005).

Exercise 7-20: *Multiple-choice question*

Warren knows that if he is able to get buy-in for this proposal, the first outcome will be:

    A. Improvement of the health status of the children

    B. Development of an action plan for improving student health

    C. Engaging teachers, parents, students, and the community in promoting health-enhancing behaviors and better health

    D. Identification of strengths and weaknesses of health promotion policies and programs

Exercise 7-21: *Fill-in*

What are the five health topics that the School Health Index (SHI) currently addresses?

1. _____

2. _____

3. _____

Answers to this chapter begin on page 181.

4. _____

5. _____

Exercise 7-22: *Fill-in*

A woman in the audience asks, "Why should schools get involved in health education? Shouldn't you be focusing on the three Rs? The school has limited finances." How should Warren respond?

_____

_____

_____

_____

Warren is successful in persuading the community to engage in the School Health Index assessment. After it is completed, two priority areas identified were nutrition and physical activity. Warren knows that diet and body weight are related to health status and that nutrition is not only important to the growth and development of children but can also reduce health risks.

Exercise 7-23: *Fill-in*

Health risks associated with poor diet include:

_____

_____

_____

_____

Warren also knows that there are many factors that influence diet and, in particular, there are some social determinants associated with diet.

Exercise 7-24: *Fill-in*

List the social determinants that affect diet and nutrition.

_____

_____

_____

_____

e   **eResource 7-9:** Warren also plans to show a video to the teachers to better understand how early intervention can help fight obesity: www.cdc.gov/CDCTV/ChildObese

Answers to this chapter begin on page 181.

Warren explains to the teachers that childhood obesity leads to significant health problems. One of the teachers asks, "What specifically are the health risks to children suffering from obesity?"

Exercise 7-25: *Select all that apply*
Childhood obesity can lead to which of the following health problems?
- ❏ Sickle cell anemia
- ❏ Heart disease
- ❏ Botulism
- ❏ Type 2 diabetes
- ❏ Asthma
- ❏ Hepatic steatosis
- ❏ Cystic fibrosis
- ❏ Sleep apnea
- ❏ Autism
- ❏ Cerebral palsy

A group of teachers who have worked with Warren previously on health promotion projects agrees to participate in this new initiative. Warren is very pleased with this.

Exercise 7-26: *Multiple-choice question*
An advantage of using an established group for health work in the community is:
- A. Goals of the project do not need to be established.
- B. The members are sure to have a commitment to the goals of the project.
- C. Group members know each other's strengths and limitations.
- D. The member will readily accept the nurse leader.

Warren uses Pender's Health Promotion Model as a guide to move forward on the initiative. He knows that the model involves several basic assumptions.

Exercise 7-27: *Select all that apply*
Pender's Health Promotion Model assumptions include:
- ❏ Individuals seek to actively regulate their own behavior.
- ❏ Individuals in all their biopsychosocial complexity interact with the environment, progressively transforming the environment and being transformed over time.
- ❏ The degree to which a family engages in health-related problem-solving and goal attainment reflects the process of family health promotion.

Answers to this chapter begin on page 181.

❑ Health professionals constitute a part of the interpersonal environment, which exerts influence on persons throughout their life span.

❑ Self-initiated reconfiguration of person-environment interactive patterns is essential to behavior change.

❑ All families possess capabilities or the health potential (strengths, motivation, resources) that serve as the basis for health promotion behavior.

Figure 7-2: Health Promotion Model

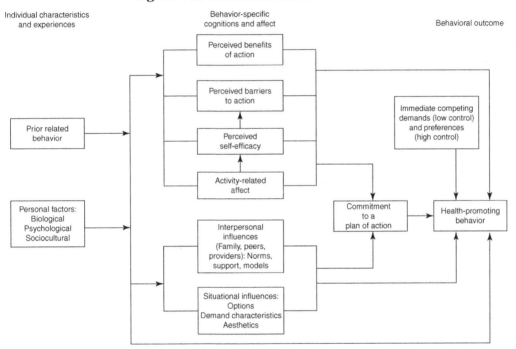

Source: Pender (1996).

Warren uses the model to start a list of strategies to move forward. He knows that he must consider and plan for a variety of factors that affect the students who are the target population.

Answers to this chapter begin on page 181.

Exercise 7-28: *Fill-in*

What should Warren plan to do to address the following identified influencing factors?

Table 7-1

Factor	Planned Approach
Personal factors	
Perceived benefits of action	
Perceived barriers to action	
Perceived self-efficacy	
Activity-related affect	
Interpersonal influences	
Situational influences	

After Warren has completed his list, he shares his ideas with the project team and asks for their input.

Answers to this chapter begin on page 181.

Answers

Exercise 7-1: *Select all that apply*

Which of the components of a typical well-child exam should Dominique expect?

☒ **Height**

☐ Head circumference

☒ **Weight**

☒ **Blood pressure**

☐ STI screening

☐ Dyslipidemia screening

☒ **Development**

☒ **BMI**

☒ **Vision test**

☒ **Hearing test**

☒ **Tuberculosis test**

Exercise 7-2: *Select all that apply*

What are the routine immunizations that should be administered to Dominique?

☒ **DTaP**

☒ **IPV**

☐ HepB

☒ **MMR**

☐ PVC

☒ **Varicella**

Exercise 7-3: *Fill-in*

Marilee knows that in addition to performing a physical assessment, it is also important for the nurse to assess for:

• **Diet and nutritional needs**

• **Elimination patterns**

• **Sleep behaviors**

• **Developmental status and behavior**

• **Safety issues**

• **Parenting concerns**

Exercise 7-4: *Multiple-choice question*

Marilee remembers Erikson's Stages of Psychosocial Development and realizes that Dominique is likely at which of the following stages:

A. Initiative versus guilt—YES, this is the Maslow's stage for preschool children.

B. Trust versus mistrust—NO, this is an earlier stage.

C. Industry versus inferiority—NO, this is later.

D. Autonomy versus shame and doubt—NO, this is later.

Exercise 7-5: *Multiple-choice question*

Marilee also realizes that at this time, Dominique is learning to:

A. Develop a sense of trust when caregivers provide reliability, care, and affection—NO, this should already have been developed.

B. Develop a sense of personal control over physical skills and a sense of independence—NO, this too is an earlier stage.

C. Develops the ability to try new things and learns how to handle failure—YES, this is part of the initiative versus guilt developmental stage.

D. Develop a sense of pride in accomplishments and abilities—NO, this will come later in school-age years.

E . Develop a sense of self and personal identity—NO, this will come later.

F . Form intimate loving relationships with other people—NO, this will come later.

Exercise 7-6: *Multiple-choice question*

By providing Tonya these materials, Marilee is engaging in which of the following:

A. Proactive education—NO, this is not the term used for teaching at this level.

B. Anticipatory guidance—YES

C. Primary prevention—NO, although it is part of primary prevention, it is more aligned with guidance and teaching.

D. Secondary prevention—NO, this is after a condition is diagnosed.

Exercise 7-7: *Multiple-choice question*

Marilee also knows that the leading cause of death for children Dominique's age is:

A. Infectious disease—NO

B. Unintentional injury—YES, so safety is the primary concern for children at this age.

C. Motor vehicle accidents—NO

D. Congenital anomalies—NO

Exercise 7-8: *Multiple-choice question*

In comparison with other high-income countries, the death rate for children under the age of 14 in the United States is ranked:

A. Among the lowest—NO

B. Third—YES

C. Fifth—NO

D. Sixth—NO

Exhibit 7-1: Answer Details

The United States ranks third with a rate of 8.7. It is surpassed by New Zealand (11.1) and Mexico (12.7). For more information, visit: http://goo.gl/MSi1Y

Exercise 7-9: *Fill-in*

What primary prevention measures can Tonya put into place to protect Dominique?

1. **Motor vehicle–related deaths: always use seat belts, child safety seats, and booster seats that are correct for a child's age and weight**

2. **Drowning: everyone should learn to swim; use a four-sided fence with self-closing and self-latching gates around the pool; and watch kids closely when they are in or around water**

3. **Poisoning: keep medicine away from children and teens; keep cleaning solutions and other toxic products in original packaging and where children can't get them**

4. **Fires and burns: use smoke alarms (where people sleep and on every level of the home and test monthly); create and practice a family fire escape plan; and install a home fire sprinkler system if possible. Kitchen safety measures**

5. **Falls: use a soft landing surface on playgrounds (such as sand or wood chips, not dirt or grass); use protective gear, like a helmet, during sports and recreation; and install protective rails on bunk beds and loft beds (CDC, April 12, 2012, p. 3)**

Exercise 7-10: *Multiple-choice question*

What would the correct response to Tonya be?

A. "Dominique doesn't need the flu shot; she is still protected by the natural immunity from breast feeding."—NO, the immunity does not protect against the flu.

B. "Dominique is young and healthy; if all of her other immunizations are up to date, she does not need the flu shot."—NO, none of the others protect against the flu.

C. "Dominique should receive the flu shot today and every year to protect her from the influenza virus."—NO, she needs a dose in 4 weeks.

D. **Dominique should receive the flu shot today and another dose in 4 weeks.—YES, this is the protocol for children.**

Exercise 7-11: *Multiple-choice question*

Before the nurse gives Dominique the flu shot, which of the following questions should she ask Tonya?

A. "Have you noticed any unusual behavior in Dominique lately?"—NO, this is not something that would affect a flu vaccine administration.

B. "Did Dominique vomit today?"—NO, the vaccine is not orally administered.

C. "When was the last time Dominique ate?"—NO, the vaccine is not orally administered.

D. "Is Dominique allergic to eggs?—YES, the vaccine is manufactured with egg protein.

Exercise 7-12: *Multiple-choice question*

What would be the best response for the nurse to give?

A. "People who get the flu shot are protected from the flu virus immediately.—NO, it takes several days to work."

B. "It takes 4 weeks (1 month) for the flu vaccination to take full effect, so if you are exposed to the flu during that time, you might get the flu."—NO, this is too long.

C. "Some illnesses have flulike symptoms, so people may mistakenly think that they have caught the flu even after getting the flu shot."—YES, this is true.

D. "Getting the flu shot can lessen the severity of illness."—YES, this is also true.

E. B and C

F. C and D

G. A, C, and D

Exercise 7-13: *True or false*

Is the influenza vaccination safe for pregnant women?

A. True—YES, because it is an attenuated virus if injected

B. False

Exercise 7-14: *Multiple-choice question*

Tonya still has questions about the flu shot and how this can affect her pregnancy. Which of the following statements made by Marilee is most accurate?

A. "The changes that occur in your body when you are pregnant build immunity against illness so you don't need the flu shot."—NO, this is not true.

B. "While pregnant women are at no greater risk from influenza as the general public, you should still get the vaccination."—NO, also not true

C. "Pregnant women with influenza are at no greater risk for premature labor than their counterparts."—NO, they are at greater risk.

D. "Getting the influenza vaccine will protect your unborn baby and protect the baby after birth."—YES, this is true because it passes the placental barrier.

E. "Since you are pregnant, it is best that you get the nasal spray flu vaccine."—NO, that is a live virus in the nasal spray.

Exercise 7-15: *Fill-in*

The National Association of School Nurses identifies seven core roles of the school nurse. List the core roles and provide a specific example of an activity for each.

1. **Direct care to students: for example, care for injuries and acute illness; long-term management of special health care needs, medication administration—asthma, diabetes mellitus, and so forth**

2. Oversight and direction for the provision of health services—disaster preparedness; plans/protocols to deal with emergencies

3. Screening—vision and hearing screening

4. Promoting a healthy school environment—monitoring immunizations

5. Promoting health—nutrition, exercise, smoking prevention and cessation

6. Leadership role for health policies and programs—health promotion and protection, chronic disease management, coordinated school health programs, school wellness policies

7. Liaison between school personnel, family, health care professionals, and the community case manager for students with health problems (Council on School Health, 2008, p. 1053)

Exercise 7-16: *Fill-in*
Identify which of the following is primary (P), secondary (S), or tertiary (T) care.

T	Health services for students with special needs
P	Health education
P	Healthful school environment
P	Physical education
T	Counseling, psychological, and social services
P	Site health promotion for faculty and staff
P, S, T	Primary care (Note: primary care addresses all levels of prevention)
T	Case management
T	Administration of medications
S	Managing minor complaints, scraps, headache, and so forth
P	Immunizations status
S	Health screening

Exercise 7-17: *Multiple-choice question*
An example of tertiary prevention that Warren provides would be:

A. Conducting screening tests or arranging for screening by others—NO, this is secondary prevention.

B. Providing first aid for a fall injury—NO, this is actual treatment and intervention.

C. Providing safety education—NO, this is primary prevention.

D. Providing for special equipment needs—YES

Exercise 7-18: *Fill-in*
Who are the key stakeholders that Warren should invite to this meeting?

Key stakeholders include parents, family, teachers, staff, local health professionals, public health representatives, city liaisons, school district representatives, interested community members.

Exercise 7-19: *Multiple-choice question*

Consensus is:

A. A unanimous vote—NO

B. A majority vote—NO, this just means over 50%.

C. Everyone 100% satisfied—NO, this is not realistic.

D. A solution that all members can support—YES

Exercise 7-20: *Multiple-choice question*

Warren knows that if he is able to get buy-in for this proposal, the first outcome will be:

A. Improvement of the health status of the children—NO, this is an outcome.

B. Development of an action plan for improving student health—NO, this is the planning stage.

C. Engaging teachers, parents, students, and the community in promoting health-enhancing behaviors and better health—NO, this is interventional.

D. Identification of strengths and weaknesses of health promotion policies and programs—YES, this will be the first step.

Exercise 7-21: *Fill-in*

What are the five health topics that the SHI currently addresses?

1. **Physical activity**
2. **Nutrition**
3. **Tobacco use prevention**
4. **Safety (unintentional injury and violence prevention)**
5. **Asthma**

Exercise 7-22: *Fill-in*

A woman in the audience asks, "Why should schools get involved in health education? Shouldn't you be focusing on the three Rs? The school has limited finances."
How should Warren respond?

Response should include:

- **Our society values good health and safety.**
- **Good health, safety, and management are necessary for effective learning.**
- **Healthy and safe students become healthy, productive citizens.**
- **Disease and injury prevention is more cost-effective than treatment. Early efforts to build healthy habits can reduce the risk for chronic diseases.**
- **The school system is the one place where most of our nation's youth can be reached.**
- **Unhealthy behaviors or poor health management can lead to heart disease, cancer, stroke, obesity, diabetes, and respiratory disease.**
- **Physical activity builds bones and muscles and helps control weight.**
- **Healthy eating helps youth grow, develop, and do well in school, allowing them to avoid obesity and eating disorders.**

- Not using tobacco promotes physical fitness, normal lung growth, and heart rate, and helps prevent respiratory symptoms.
- Preventing unintentional injuries works to eliminate the leading causes of death and disability among young people.
- Effective asthma management can reduce hospitalization and school absences, leading to a healthier and more productive lifestyle (CDC, 2005, pp. 15–16).

Exercise 7-23: *Fill-in*

Health risks associated with poor diet include:

- **Overweight and obesity**
- **Malnutrition**
- **Iron-deficiency anemia**
- **Heart disease**
- **High blood pressure**
- **Dyslipidemia (poor lipid profiles)**
- **Type 2 diabetes**
- **Osteoporosis**
- **Oral disease**
- **Constipation**
- **Diverticular disease**
- **Some cancers**

(U.S. Department of Health and Human Services [HHS], Healthy People 2020, 2012)

Exercise 7-24: *Fill-in*

List the social determinants that affect diet and nutrition.

Social factors thought to influence diet include:

- **Knowledge and attitudes**
- **Skills**
- **Social support**
- **Societal and cultural norms**
- **Food and agricultural policies**
- **Food assistance programs**
- **Economics—cost of living/food**

Exercise 7-25: *Select all that apply*

Childhood obesity can lead to which of the following health problems:

☒ **Sickle cell anemia**

☒ **Heart disease**

☐ Botulism

☒ **Type 2 diabetes**

☒ **Asthma**

☒ **Hepatic steatosis**

☒ **Cystic fibrosis**

☒ **Sleep apnea**

❏ Autism

❏ Cerebral palsy

Exercise 7-26: *Multiple-choice question*

An advantage of using an established group for health work in the community is:

  A. Goals of the project do not need to be established.—NO, goals are needed in order for all to understand the purpose.

  B. The members are sure to have a commitment to the goals of the project.—NO, this may not be true.

  C. Group members know each other's strengths and limitations.—YES

  D. The member will readily accept the nurse leader.—NO, this may not be true also.

Exercise 7-27: *Select all that apply*

Pender's Health Promotion Model assumptions include:

☒ **Individuals seek to actively regulate their own behavior.**

☒ **Individuals in all their biopsychosocial complexity interact with the environment, progressively transforming the environment and being transformed over time.**

❏ The degree to which a family engages in health-related problem-solving and goal attainment reflects the process of family health promotion.

☒ **Health professionals constitute a part of the interpersonal environment, which exerts influence on persons throughout their life span.**

☒ **Self-initiated reconfiguration of person-environment interactive patterns is essential to behavior change.**

❏ All families possess capabilities or the health potential (strengths, motivation, resources) that serve as the basis for health promotion behavior (NursingPlanet. com, 2012, p. 3).

Exercise 7-28: *Fill-in*

What should Warren plan to do to address the following identified influencing factors?

Table 7-2

Factor	Planned Approach
Personal factors	**Personal factors categorized as** • **Biological: need to accommodate all levels of ability** • **Psychological: consider self-esteem, self-motivation, and confidence in ability to change** • **Sociocultural: race ethnicity, acculturation, education, and socioeconomic status**
Perceived benefits of action	**Students need to believe/anticipate that there will be a positive outcome of changing behavior**
Perceived barriers to action	**Need to anticipate any real or imagined barriers and put into place measures to remove, address proactively, and minimize effect of barrier(s)**
Perceived self-efficacy	**Assess perceptions of personal capability to establish and implement a health-promoting behavior; measures to build self-efficacy capacity**
Activity-related affect	**Anticipate what measures can make health behavior a positive and fun experience; generate social engagement/excitement; student "team leaders"; local celebrities; focus on feeling good after physical activity**
Interpersonal influences	**Leverage strengths and influences from interpersonal relationships such as established norms, social support, and modeling desired behavior. Keep in mind the primary sources of interpersonal influences are families, peers, and health care providers**
Situational influences	**Anticipate situational/environmental influences; can activity take place in a safe and comfortable environment?**

8

Community Health Programs

Unfolding Case Study #1 ▬ Cultural Competence

Sadie Galloway is a nurse working in an underserved community in a medium-sized urban city in New York State. The community she serves has large Hispanic and Asian communities. She understands that she must be aware of her own personal cultural values and beliefs when working with clients from different cultures.

Exercise 8-1: *Multiple-choice question*
Cultural competence is best defined as:

    A. The process in which the health care professional seeks and obtains a sound educational base about culturally diverse groups (Lavizzo-Mourey, 1996)

    B. The process of conducting a self-examination of one's own biases toward other cultures and the in-depth exploration of one's cultural and professional background (Campinha-Bacote, 2002)

    C. An ongoing process that involves accepting and respecting differences and not letting one's personal beliefs have an undue influence on those whose worldview is different from one's own and includes having general cultural as well as cultural-specific information (Giger et al., 2007)

    D. The ability to conduct a cultural assessment to collect relevant cultural data regarding the client's presenting problem as well as accurately conducting a culturally based physical assessment (Campinha-Bacote, 2002)

Sadie also knows that she must consider a variety of factors when providing culturally competent care.

Exercise 8-2: *Fill-in*
Which factors must be considered when providing culturally competent care?

_____

_____

_____

_____

Answers to this chapter begin on page 210.

Sadie remembers learning about Giger and Davidhizar's (1991) Transcultural Assessment Model, which provides a transcultural nursing perspective when conducting an assessment or planning nursing interventions. The Transcultural Assessment Model considers the diversity of the individual from six areas.

Exercise 8-3: *Fill-in*

List the six areas of human diversity considered in the Transcultural Assessment Model:

1. _____

2. _____

3. _____

4. _____

5. _____

6. _____

Exercise 8-4: *Multiple-choice question*

Which of the following terms examines our beliefs and values as they influence behavior?

    A. Cultural knowledge

    B. Cultural skill

    C. Cultural awareness

    D. Cultural encounter

Sadie's colleague, Bernard, believes strongly that the best approach to providing quality, equitable health care to all individuals is to treat all of his clients the same no matter what cultural group the person belongs to. "We should approach it like Lady Justice and be blind to those differences." Sadie knows that what Bernard is describing is termed "cultural blindness."

Exercise 8-5: *Multiple-choice question*

Cultural blindness is best defined as:

    A. When all individuals, no matter what race, ethnicity, or cultural affinity, receive care that reflects sensitivity and appreciation for the diversity of another

    B. The belief that cultural differences are of little importance and care or treatments traditionally used by the dominant culture are believed to be universally applicable to all groups

    C. Treatment of a person based upon the group, class, or category to which that person belongs rather than upon the individual

    D. Accommodation to certain cultural characteristics, values, belief systems, history, and behaviors of the members of another ethnic group

Answers to this chapter begin on page 210.

Exercise 8-6: *Fill-in*

Discuss the pros and cons of cultural blindness when working with a diverse population.

_____

_____

_____

_____

Exercise 8-7: *Select all that apply*

Culturally competent health care is reflected by:

❑ Awareness of personal culture, values, beliefs, and behaviors

❑ Knowledge of and respect for different cultures

❑ Skills in interacting with and responding to individuals from other cultures

❑ Treatment of a person based upon the group, class, or category to which that person belongs rather than upon the individual

❑ Acknowledgment of the importance of culture and its incorporation at all levels

❑ Assessment of cross-cultural relations

❑ Vigilance toward the dynamics that result from cultural differences and expansion of cultural knowledge

❑ Provision of services to meet universal health care needs

Exercise 8-8: *Matching*

Match the term in Column A to the correct definition in Column B.

Column A	Column B
A. Stereotyping	_____ Treatment or consideration of a person based upon the group, class, or category to which that person belongs rather than upon the individual
B. Discrimination	_____ A psychological disorientation that most people experience when living in a culture significantly different from their own
C. Acculturation	_____ Occurs when one applies the majority cultural perspective or norm to individuals and families; such as prescribing a special diet without regard to the client's culture

Answers to this chapter begin on page 210.

Column A	Column B
D. Prejudice	_____ The process of incorporating some of the cultural attributes of the larger society by diverse groups, individuals, or peoples
E. Cultural awareness	_____ The preconception that members of one race are intrinsically superior to members of other races
F. Racism	_____ A learned, patterned behavioral response acquired over time that includes implicit versus explicit beliefs, attitudes, values, customs, norms, taboos, arts, and life ways accepted by a community of individuals
G. Ethnocentrism	_____ The process by which people acquire and recall information about others based on race, sex, religion, and so forth
H. Cultural shock	_____ Irrational suspicion or hatred of a particular group, race, or religion
I. Diversity	_____ Experienced when neutral language—both verbal and nonverbal—is used in a way that reflects sensitivity and appreciation for the diversity of another
J. Cultural imposition	_____ Being knowledgeable about one's own thoughts, feelings, and sensations, as well as the ability to reflect on how these can affect one's interactions with others
K. Culture	_____ Differences in the incidence, prevalence, mortality, and burden of disease and other adverse health conditions that exist among specific population groups in the United States
L. Cultural sensitivity	_____ An all-inclusive concept, and includes differences in race, color, ethnicity, national origin, and immigration status, religion, age, gender, sexual orientation, ability or disability, and other attributes of groups of people in society
M. Health disparity	_____ Arise because of the differences in values and norms of behavior of people from different cultures
N. Cultural conflict	_____ When a person acts on prejudice and denies another person one or more of his or her fundamental rights (American Association of Colleges of Nursing, 2008)

Answers to this chapter begin on page 210.

Exercise 8-9: *Multiple-choice question*

Sadie understands that culture has an effect on a person's behavior and that it is important to consider culture when providing health care or health education because:

    A. Culture is part of one's genetic traits and cannot be altered

    B. All members of a cultural group have similar responses to health interventions

    C. Culture includes learned behaviors and beliefs transmitted by the family, ethnic group, and society

    D. Determines the client's ability for self-care in response to disease or illness

Sadie also knows that being culturally competent involves attention to culturally sensitive communication and that communication involves verbal as well as non-verbal communication.

Exercise 8-10: *Multiple-choice question*

She remembers that it is important to keep in mind that:

    A. Anglo-Americans tend to prefer formal verbal communication

    B. Using terms of endearment such as "honey" or "sweetie" helps establish rapport with clients

    C. Engaging in "small talk" and asking personal questions helps in establishing a relationship with clients

    D. Asking clients how they would like to be addressed helps in establishing rapport

Bernard remembers the Campinha-Bacote Model of Cultural Competence that he learned about in school. He tells Sadie that according to this model, individuals and organizations must first demonstrate a motivation to be culturally competent before moving toward achieving cultural competence.

Exercise 8-11: *Multiple-choice question*

According to Campinha-Bacote (2008), cultural skill is when a nurse:

    A. Becomes "sensitive to the values, beliefs, lifestyle, and practices of the patient/client, and explores her/his own values, biases and prejudices"

    B. Understands the "values, beliefs, practices, and problem-solving strategies of culturally/ethnically diverse groups"

    C. Is able to "conduct a cultural assessment in partnership with the client/patient"

    D. Engages in "cross-cultural interactions with people who are culturally/ethnically diverse from oneself"

Answers to this chapter begin on page 210.

eResource 8-1: Both Bernard and Sadie are interested in becoming more culturally competent and better able to work effectively in cross-cultural situations. To improve their skills, the two sign up for free training: http://goo.gl/CkRLc

Both Sadie and Bernard learned a lot from the training. They decide to share two brief videos that highlight the importance of culturally and linguistically appropriate services with their colleagues at the agency.

 eResource 8-2: Health Equity & Culturally and Linguistically Appropriate Services (CLAS):
■ Think–Speak–Act Cultural Health: Part 1: http://goo.gl/q091n
■ Think–Speak–Act Cultural Health: Part 2: http://goo.gl/8qT0w

Exercise 8-12: *Select all that apply*
Factors to consider in nonverbal communication include:
- ❑ Silence
- ❑ Socioeconomic status
- ❑ Distance
- ❑ Physical attributes
- ❑ Eye contact
- ❑ Emotional or facial expression
- ❑ Dietary preferences
- ❑ Body positioning
- ❑ Gestures
- ❑ Touch

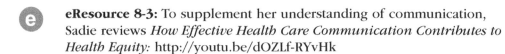 **eResource 8-3:** To supplement her understanding of communication, Sadie reviews *How Effective Health Care Communication Contributes to Health Equity:* http://youtu.be/dOZLf-RYvHk

Sadie knows that if she will be preparing health education materials, she needs to make sure that the materials are culturally appropriate and that the *form* of the material is just as important as the *content*.

Exercise 8-13: *Select all that apply*
The *form* of the health education material refers to:
- ❑ Concepts
- ❑ Style
- ❑ Vocabulary
- ❑ Perspective
- ❑ Voice
- ❑ Story line

Answers to this chapter begin on page 210.

Exercise 8-14: *True or false*

In addition, Sadie knows she must make sure that materials she develops must be readable. The *readability* of a document refers to the ease with which the eye can recognize words on a document.

    A. True

    B. False

Exercise 8-15: *Fill-in*

Sadie realizes that health education materials must be readable. Strategies to ensure readability of patient education materials include:

1. _____

2. _____

3. _____

4. _____

5. _____

6. _____

7. _____

8. _____

e   **eResource 8-4:** Sadie uses the CDC's publication *Simply Put: A Guide for Creating Easy-to-Understand Materials* as a resource to help prepare her educational materials: http://goo.gl/L9SNf

Exercise 8-16: *Select all that apply*

Sadie knows that putting time into ensuring the health education materials she creates are clear, to the point, and readable will have the following benefits:

    ❑ Reaches people who cannot read well or who don't have time to read well

    ❑ Reduces health care costs

    ❑ Helps all readers understand information

    ❑ Meets the needs of all community members

    ❑ Avoids misunderstandings and errors

    ❑ Avoids confusion

    ❑ Saves time because it gets the job done well the first time

Sadie and Bernard decide to review all the patient education materials used by their office to determine the level of readability and identify any need for modification of these materials. They decide to use two tools to complete this assessment: SMOG and Fry Readability tools.

Answers to this chapter begin on page 210.

Exercise 8-17: *Fill-in*

Select a patient education document/pamphlet of your choice and use the SMOG and Fry Readability tools to conduct a readability analysis and compare results.

 eResource 8-5: If the material is available electronically, use
- McLaughlin's free online SMOG Readability (Simple Measure of Gobbledygook) tool: http://goo.gl/ulEy5
- ATOS Readability Tool from Renaissance Learning: http://goo.gl/DQkr3

Exercise 8-18: *Fill-in*

If the material is only available in hard copy, use Appendix C of *Simply Put* (http://goo.gl/L9SNf) to do the analysis. Do the two tools provide the same readability score?

SMOG: _____

_____

Fry: _____

_____

Bernard and Sadie want to add to their library of patient education materials, so they begin to look at various governmental and nonprofit websites to see what is available. They are particularly interested in locating resources that provide culturally appropriate materials. Bernard finds two resources that he bookmarks for future access.

 eResource 8-6: Culturally appropriate patient education materials:
- EthnoMed: http://ethnomed.org/patient-education
- Health Information Translations: www.healthinfotranslations.org

Unfolding Case Study #2 ▨ Community Assessment

Sadie wants to get a better understanding of the community, so she decides to do a community assessment. Sadie reflects on the concept of community. She remembers that community can be defined very broadly.

Exercise 8-19: *Fill-in*

What is the definition of a "community"?

_____

_____

_____

_____

Answers to this chapter begin on page 210.

Her first step is to do a windshield survey that will provide her with an initial overview of the community.

Exercise 8-20: *Multiple-choice question*
A windshield survey is all of the following except:
    A. A composite of subjective and objective data that help define a community
    B. Contains information about trends, stability, and changes that will affect the health of the population
    C. Is always conducted while the observer sits in a car
    D. Provides a visual overview of a community. A person can also perform a windshield survey by walking through the targeted area
    E. Relies on observations for data and other information instead of directing questions to participants

Sadie also knows that when doing a windshield survey, she should be looking at key aspects within the community.

Exercise 8-21: *Fill-in*
List the components of a windshield survey:

_____

_____

_____

_____

_____

Sadie remembers that in addition to the information collected while doing a windshield survey, she also needs to collect information from other resources. She knows that these sources can be categorized as primary data and secondary data.

Exercise 8-22: *Fill-in*
Primary data sources include:

_____

_____

_____

_____

Answers to this chapter begin on page 210.

Secondary data sources include:

_____

_____

_____

_____

Sadie knows that resources to provide community programs and services are limited, and therefore it is essential that community assessments are accurate. She wants to make sure that the assessment she does correctly identifies the major areas of concern, the populations at risk, and the types of interventions that may have a positive health outcome. To supplement her understanding of the steps involved in a comprehensive community assessment, Sadie watches a video produced by the New York State Department of Health.

 eResource 8-7: Community Health Assessment: Finding the Information You Need: http://vimeo.com/36837196

Sadie decides to conduct interviews and focus groups to collect additional information about the community and community needs.

Exercise 8-23: *Multiple-choice question*
Conducting interviews is considered:
       A. Rapport building
       B. Culturally sensitive
       C. Primary data collection
       D. Secondary data collection

Sadie knows that there are additional resources for secondary data. These include United States Census Data and Vital Statistics. In addition, she looks for other sources of data to ensure a comprehensive assessment.

 eResource 8-8: Sadie notices that there is a public library just within the boundaries of the community she is assessing. She knows that the public libraries use the statistics from the U.S. Census, so she consults the Public Library Geographic Database (PLGDB): http://goo.gl/qgDPw

Sadie's colleague, Bernard, shows her some additional data sources to supplement the data she has already collected.

 eResource 8-9: To locate additional information regarding health statistics data for infants, children, adolescents, adults, and older adults, Bernard accesses
    ■ The CDC's Interactive Health Data site: http://goo.gl/ObwJD
    ■ The Health Indicators website: http://healthindicators.gov/

Unfolding Case Study #3 — Community Partnerships to Improve Health Outcomes

Sadie is also responsible for working with various constituencies in the community to plan and provide health education programs. Her superiors have encouraged her to utilize Healthy People 2020 goals for the health of Americans. She realizes that Healthy People 2020 is an evidence-based approach to improving health outcomes.

Exercise 8-24: *Fill-in*
What are the overarching goals of Healthy People 2020?

1. _____

2. _____

3. _____

4. _____

Exercise 8-25: *Fill-in*
What is health disparity?

_____

_____

 eResource 8-10: To better understand the focus of Healthy People 2020, Sadie also views the video *Preparing for the Next Decade: A 2020 Vision for Healthy People*: http://youtu.be/zZG94c7xQmE

Exercise 8-26: *Multiple-choice question*
When Sadie plans culturally appropriate health education programs for the community, which of the following strategies should she use?

    A. Set goals that reflect mainstream values

    B. Consult with local groups, leaders, and individuals

    C. Use all available communication methods to get the message out

    D. Consider using health care experts to deliver the message

Sadie is invited to do a presentation at a Parent-Teachers Organization (PTO) meeting. She decides to approach the presentation from a broad community health perspective using Healthy People 2020's overarching goals and health determinants as a foundation to generate interest in community approaches to improve health. Sadie recalls what she knows about health determinants.

Answers to this chapter begin on page 210.

Exercise 8-27: *True or false*

For the most part, individuals have direct control over all their health determinants and can take steps to improve their own health.

    A. True

    B. False

Exercise 8-28: *Select all that apply*

Determinants of health are:

    ❏ The economic factors impacting individuals or populations

    ❏ The physical environment impacting individuals or populations

    ❏ A person's individual characteristics and behaviors

    ❏ A person's genetic makeup

    ❏ The social factors impacting individuals or populations

Sadie opens her presentation by thanking the leadership and members of the PTO for inviting her to speak. She provides an overview of her role in the community. Sadie tells the members of the community, "Health is not just something we get at the doctor's office. Health starts in our families, in our schools and workplaces, in our playgrounds and parks. The more we see the problem of health this way, the more opportunities we have to improve it. The conditions in which we live and work have an enormous impact on our health, long before we ever see a doctor. Factors such as income, education, and child development have a profound impact on health" (Wellington-Dufferin-Guelph Public Health, 2012, p. 1).

 eResource 8-11: To start the conversation about strategies that can be implemented to help improve the health of the community, Sadie shows the group a brief video, *Let's Start a Conversation About Health . . . and Not Talk About Health Care at All:* http://youtu.be/jbqKcOqoyoo

The video generates good discussion among the group. But some of the residents seem to be overwhelmed. "How do we begin?" asks one person, "Some of these problems are really big and I don't see how our small group can make any difference." Sadie replies, "Let's break it down to make it more manageable." Sadie provides several scenarios that highlight the benefit of community health interventions that can have an impact upon determinants of health.

 eResource 8-12: To drive home this idea, Sadie shows the group a video, *Healthy People 2020—Determinants of Health:* http://youtu.be/5Yb3B75eqbo

Answers to this chapter begin on page 210.

After the presentation, Sadie reviews scenarios that highlighted the benefit of community health interventions that can have an impact upon determinants of health. "Let's start by talking about the little girl, Carla, who was in the video. What measures were put into place to help impact her health determinants?"

Exercise 8-29: *Fill-in*
What measures were put into place to help impact Carla's health determinants?

_____

_____

_____

Sadie then engages the group in a brainstorming activity. "Let's talk about what is important to you and your community. Frequently a group will come up with a list of areas of concern. This exercise is designed to help you identify these and then prioritize."

 eResource 8-13: Sadie hands out a document to each attendee and asks them to work in small groups to discuss the guiding questions regarding setting priorities: http://goo.gl/E7yqC

After extensive discussion, the group identifies two priority areas in which they would like to see improvement:
1. Need for opportunities for physical activity in safe and supervised settings
2. Underage drinking

"The next step," Sadie tells the members of the PTO, "is to identify our community assets. Community assets are strengths and resources within the community that can partner with you to help achieve your goals. So let's brainstorm a bit about available resources within our community."

 eResource 8-14: Sadie provides the group with another handout that lists potential resources that can serve as "cues" for brainstorming: http://goo.gl/L1IgX

Sadie leaves the meeting energized and excited about being involved in this coalition. She knows that the next steps involve continuing to assess and identify not only community assets but also the potential barriers. The next is to bring together the community members with the key stakeholders in the community to build consensus and develop a plan that is feasible and effective. In addition, there must be a way to measure the program's effectiveness—specifically, its impact upon health outcomes.

Sadie also begins to look for additional resources that can help with collecting information as well as provide tools to address the priority areas identified.

Figure 8-1: Prioritizing Issues Exercise

Exercise: Prioritizing Issues

Healthy People 2020

Likelihood of success/impact (taking into account available resources): _____

Current interventions addressing issue in community: _____

Consequences if not addressed (personal, societal, economic): _____

Healthy People 2020

Exercise:

Prioritizing Issues

ASSESS

Coalition members will likely have many issues they want to address. This exercise is designed to help the group decide which issue(s) to focus on.

First, make a list of all the issues on the table. Then, working as a group, copy and complete this sheet for each issue you are considering. Use the information to help narrow down your target issue(s).

Issue: _____

Prevalence/frequency/incidence: _____

Population(s) affected: _____

Seriousness/urgency: _____

Available data sources: _____

Possible interventions (behavioral, environmental, legislative, etc.): _____

Source: Adapted from *Healthy People 2010 Toolkit: A Field Guide to Health Planning.* Developed by the Public Health Foundation, under contract with the Office of Disease Prevention and Health Promotion, Office of Public Health and Science, U.S. Department of Health and Human Services (pp. 74–75). Available: http://healthypeople.gov/2020/implementing/assess.apsx

Answers to this chapter begin on page 210.

Figure 8-2: Evaluation of Community Strengths

ASSESS

Brainstorm:

Community Assets

Healthy People 2020

Work with your planning group to create a list of potential assets in your community. It's important to take stock of the strengths of your community, not just its needs. Community assets are important in three ways:

- As inputs and context for your public health intervention
- As factors related to successful implementation of your intervention
- As potential outputs, signaling the impact of your intervention

Use the list below to help guide your brainstorm of community strengths.

Individuals

- Skills, talents, and experience of community members
- Individual businesses
- Home-based enterprises
- Donations/financial sponsors

Organizations

- Associations of businesses
- Citizens' associations
- Cultural organizations
- Communications organizations
- Faith-based organizations

Private and Nonprofit Organizations

- Institutions of higher education
- Hospitals
- Social services agencies

Public Institutions and Services

- Public schools
- Police and fire departments
- Libraries
- Parks and recreation

Physical Resources

- Vacant land
- Commercial and industrial structures
- Housing
- Energy and waste resources
- Billboards and community bulletin boards
- Community meeting spaces

Informal Organizations and "Intangibles"

- Neighborhood associations and other social groups
- Community reputation
- Community pride

Source: Healthy People 2020 Tools. Available: http://healthypeople.gov/2020/implementing/assess.apsx

Answers to this chapter begin on page 210.

Of particular importance is collecting data that support the need to provide programs. To support requests for underage drinking prevention programing, Sadie knows she must demonstrate the impact this undesired behavior is having by documenting the costs associated with underage drinking.

 eResource 8-15: Sadie accesses and reviews resources made available by focusing particular attention on the costs associated with underage drinking [Pathway: www.udetc.org → select "Underage Drinking Costs" → use drop-down box to select your State information]

As she prepares for her next community meeting, Sadie reviews materials she received sometime ago that addressed the community assessment process.

 eResource 8-16: *Community Needs Assessment: Models and Measurements*: http://goo.gl/YgGnD; and *Conducting a Community Assessment*: http://goo.gl/hKjqu

Reviewing this resource underscored the value of community and key stakeholder involvement and the importance of using a model to guide development of this community-based initiative. So Sadie considers a variety of models to provide structure to the planned program.

Exercise 8-30: *Matching*
Match the model in Column A with the correct description in Column B.

Column A	Column B
A. PRECEDE-PROCEED Model	_____ Serves as a data collection tool and planning resource for community members who want to make their community a healthier one
B. PATCH Model	_____ Incorporates systems thinking, which involves examining the underlying structure of community health issues and systems in order to create lasting positive change on a community level
C. MAPP	_____ Premise is that a change process should focus initially on the outcome, not on the activity; it is a participatory process, involving those affected by the issue or condition
D. CHANGE	_____ Process that many communities use to collect and use local data, set health priorities, plan, conduct, and evaluate health promotion and disease prevention programs

Answers to this chapter begin on page 210.

Exhibit 8-1: Snapshot of Action Steps for Completing the CHANGE Tool

The following is a summary of the action steps that are suggested for successfully completing the CHANGE tool.

ACTION STEP 1: Assemble the Community Team

Identify and assemble the community team; diverse representation is preferred. Consider the makeup of the team to include 10 to 12 individuals maximum.

ACTION STEP 2: Develop Team Strategy

Decide whether to complete CHANGE as a whole team or divide into subgroups. Communities tend to divide the team into subgroups, ensuring there are two people collecting and analyzing data and reporting back to the team to gain consensus.

ACTION STEP 3: Review All 5 CHANGE Sectors

Review all five sectors prior to completing them, so the community team understands the total picture of what is being assessed. These include the (a) Community-at-Large Sector, (b) Community Institution or Organization (CIO) Sector, (c) Health Care Sector, (d) School Sector, and (e) Work Site Sector.

ACTION STEP 4: Gather Data

Use multiple methods (two or more) to gather data from each site to maximize the data quality. Methods could include, for example, focus groups, windshield surveys, or questionnaires. Consider the amount of time needed for each of the methods selected.

ACTION STEP 5: Review Data Gathered

Gather with the community team to review the data received. Brainstorm, debate, and dialogue with the team to gain consensus on what these data mean in terms of parameters of the CHANGE tool. Data should be rated based on a comprehensive review of all sources and agreement of everyone involved.

ACTION STEP 6: Enter Data

Use the CHANGE Sector Excel File to enter data. Within the community team, make sure there is a designated data manager to input the data. Complete a separate CHANGE Sector Excel File for each site.

(continued)

Answers to this chapter begin on page 210.

Exhibit 8-1: Snapshot of Action Steps for Completing the CHANGE Tool (*continued*)

ACTION STEP 7: Review Consolidated Data

Once ratings have been assigned to each sector, the following steps will need to be completed so the team can begin to determine areas of improvement to develop a Community Action Plan based on the community-level data.

ACTION STEP 7a: Create a CHANGE Summary Statement

ACTION STEP 7b: Complete the Sector Data Grid

ACTION STEP 7c: Fill out the CHANGE Strategy Worksheets

ACTION STEP 7d: Complete the Community Health Improvement Planning Template

ACTION STEP 8: Build the Community Action Plan

The final step is to build a Community Action Plan. This will be organized by project period and annual objectives, and reflect the data collected during the CHANGE process.

Source: CDC Healthy Communities Program: Community Health Assessment and Group Evaluation (CHANGE). Available: http://www.cdc.gov/healthycommunitiesprogram/tools/change/pdf/changeactionguide.pdf

Answers to this chapter begin on page 210.

Sadie realizes that even though the members of the PTO were very enthusiastic about moving forward on efforts to improve the health of the community, it is important that all members of the community have an opportunity to be involved in the assessment and planning process. The handout for Brainstorming for Community Assets was very helpful in identifying other parties to involve. She discusses next steps with her colleague Bernard. They decide to invite all parties to a meeting. After discussion, they determine that the CHANGE model as a framework to move forward would work well. The key agenda item would be to assemble a team.

 eResource 8-17: Bernard locates additional information about the Community Health Assessment and Group Evaluation (CHANGE) project: Guideline Manual: http://goo.gl/2j503

Sadie and Bernard decide that they will want to publicize the program. They realize that it is too early to do that, but also want to make sure that they are properly prepared when the time comes. They know that it is important for them to use the media effectively to get the health message out. They also realize that they need some guidance in determining what social media tools best meet their needs.

 eResource 8-18: Bernard locates *The Health Communicators Social Media Toolkit*, a resource from the CDC that can help them get started: http://goo.gl/x6xcD

Answers to this chapter begin on page 210.

Answers

Exercise 8-1: *Multiple-choice question*

Cultural competence is best defined as:

A. The process in which the health care professional seeks and obtains a sound educational base about culturally diverse groups (Lavizzo-Mourey, 1996)—NO, education alone is not enough.

B. The process of conducting a self-examination of one's own biases toward other cultures and the in-depth exploration of one's cultural and professional background (Campinha-Bacote, 2002)—NO, this is helpful, but again it is not enough alone.

C. An ongoing process that involves accepting and respecting differences and not letting one's personal beliefs have an undue influence on those whose worldview is different from one's own and includes having general cultural as well as cultural-specific information (Giger et al., 2007)—YES

D. The ability to conduct a cultural assessment to collect relevant cultural data regarding the client's presenting problem as well as accurately conducting a culturally based physical assessment (Campinha-Bacote, 2002)—NO, self-reflection is also needed.

Exercise 8-2: *Fill-in*

Which factors must be considered when providing culturally competent care?

- **Race**
- **Social class**
- **Socioeconomic**
- **Religion**
- **Ethnicity**
- **Education**
- **Language**
- **Literacy**
- **Health literacy**
- **Environment**

Exercise 8-3: *Fill-in*

Exhibit 8-2: Giger and Davidhizar's Transcultural Assessment Model

1. **Communication.** The factors that influence communication are universal, but vary among culture-specific groups in terms of language spoken, voice quality, pronunciation, use of silence, and use of nonverbal communication.
2. **Space.** People perceive physical and personal space through their biological senses. The cultural aspect of space is in determining the degree of comfort one feels in proximity to others, in body movement, and in perception of personal, intimate, and public space.
3. **Social Orientation.** Components of social organization vary by culture, with differences observed in what constitutes one's understanding of culture, race, ethnicity, family role and function, work, leisure, church, and friends in day-to-day life.
4. **Time.** Time is perceived, measured, and valued differently across cultures. Time is conceptualized in reference to the life span in terms of growth and developments, perception of time in relation to duration of events, and time as an external entity, outside our control.
5. **Environmental Control.** Environment is more than just the place where one lives, and involves systems and processes that influence and are influenced by individuals and groups. Culture shapes an understanding of how individuals and groups shape their environments and how environments constrain or enable individual health behaviors.
6. **Biological Variations.** The need to understand the biological variations is necessary in order to avoid generalizations and stereotyping behavior. Biological variations are dimensions such as body structure, body weight, skin color, internal biological mechanisms such as genetic and enzymatic predisposition to certain diseases, drug interactions, and metabolism. (American Association of Colleges of Nursing, August 2008, p. 6)

Exercise 8-4: *Multiple-choice question*

Which of the following terms examines our beliefs and values as they influence behavior?

A. Cultural knowledge—NO, this only assesses the cognitive domain.
B. Cultural skill—NO, this only assesses the psychomotor and cognitive domains.
C. **Cultural awareness—YES, this assesses the affective domain of learning.**
D. Cultural encounter—NO, this only assesses the psychomotor and cognitive domains if not reflected on afterward.

Exercise 8-5: *Multiple-choice question*

Cultural blindness is best defined as:

A. When all individuals, no matter what race, ethnicity, or cultural affinity, receive care that reflects sensitivity and appreciation for the diversity of another—NO, this is cultural awareness.

B. **The belief that cultural differences are of little importance and care or treatments traditionally used by the dominant culture are believed to be universally applicable to all groups—YES**

C. Treatment of a person based upon the group, class, or category to which that person belongs rather than on the individual—NO, this is cultural stereotyping.

D. Accommodation to certain cultural characteristics, values, belief systems, history, and behaviors of the members of another ethnic group—NO, this is cultural awareness.

Exercise 8-6: *Fill-in*

Discuss the pros and cons of cultural blindness when working with a diverse population.

While on the surface, cultural blindness seems an ideal to strive for, it is not. This perspective assumes that everyone is the same . . . and we are not. This perspective discounts the individual differences. Everyone is influenced by culture. Not recognizing that there are differences among and between cultures or believing that cultural differences are not important is problematic. Cultural blindness results in a failure to consider cultural differences when providing health care.

Exercise 8-7: *Select all that apply*

Culturally competent health care is reflected by:

☒ **Awareness of personal culture, values, beliefs, and behaviors.**

☒ **Knowledge of and respect for different cultures.**

☒ **Skills in interacting with and responding to individuals from other cultures.**

❑ Treatment of a person based upon the group, class, or category to which that person belongs rather than on the individual.

☒ **Acknowledgment of the importance of culture and its incorporation at all levels.**

☒ **Assessment of cross-cultural relations.**

☒ **Vigilance toward the dynamics that result from cultural differences and expansion of cultural knowledge.**

❑ Provision of services to meet universal health care needs.

Exercise 8-8: *Matching*

Match the term in Column A with the correct definition in Column B.

Column A		Column B
A. Stereotyping	**B**	Treatment or consideration of a person based upon the group, class, or category to which that person belongs rather than on the individual
B. Discrimination	**H**	A psychological disorientation that most people experience when living in a culture significantly different from their own
C. Acculturation	**K**	Occurs when one applies the majority cultural perspective or norm to individual and families; such as prescribing a special diet without regard to the client's culture
D. Prejudice	**C**	The process of incorporating some of the cultural attributes of the larger society by diverse groups, individuals, or peoples
E. Cultural awareness	**F**	The preconception that members of one race are intrinsically superior to members of other races
F. Racism	**L**	A learned, patterned behavioral response acquired over time that includes implicit versus explicit beliefs, attitudes, values, customs, norms, taboos, arts, and life ways accepted by a community of individuals
G. Ethnocentrism	**A**	The process by which people acquire and recall information about others based on race, sex, religion, and so forth
H. Cultural shock	**D**	Irrational suspicion or hatred of a particular group, race, or religion
I. Diversity	**L**	Experienced when neutral language—both verbal and nonverbal—is used in a way that reflects sensitivity and appreciation for the diversity of another
J. Cultural imposition	**E**	Being knowledgeable about one's own thoughts, feelings, and sensations, as well as the ability to reflect on how these can affect one's interactions with others
K. Culture	**M**	Differences in the incidence, prevalence, mortality, and burden of disease and other adverse health conditions that exist among specific population groups in the United States
L. Cultural sensitivity	**I**	An all-inclusive concept, and includes differences in race, color, ethnicity, national origin, and immigration status, religion, age, gender, sexual orientation, ability/disability, and other attributes of groups of people in society

Column A		Column B
M. Health disparity	__N__	Arise because of the differences in values and norms of behavior of people from different cultures
N. Cultural conflict	__B__	When a person acts on prejudice and denies another person one or more of his or her fundamental rights (American Association of Colleges of Nursing, 2008)

Exercise 8-9: *Multiple-choice question*

Sadie understands that culture has an effect on a person's behavior and that it is important to consider culture when providing health care or health education because:

A. Culture is part of one's genetic traits and cannot be altered—NO, culture is learned, not passed down as heredity.

B. All members of a cultural group have similar responses to health interventions—NO, they will not.

C. Culture includes learned behaviors and beliefs transmitted by the family, ethnic group, and society—YES

D. Determines the client's ability for self-care in response to disease or illness—NO, other variables also need to be considered.

Exercise 8-10: *Multiple-choice question*

She remembers that it is important to keep in mind that:

A. Anglo-Americans tend to prefer formal verbal communication—NO, this is not enough to establish a rapport.

B. Using terms of endearment such as "honey" or "sweetie" helps establish rapport with clients—NO, this may be insulting to some.

C. Engaging in "small talk" and asking personal questions help in establishing a relationship with clients—NO, this is not enough to establish a rapport and may seem to some that you are ignoring the issues.

D. Asking clients how they would like to be addressed helps in establishing rapport—YES, this is polite and respectful.

Exercise 8-11: *Multiple-choice question*

According to Campinha-Bacote (2008), cultural skill is when a nurse:

A. Becomes "sensitive to the values, beliefs, lifestyle, and practices of the patient/client, and explores her/his own values, biases and prejudices"—NO, this is cultural awareness.

B. Understands the "values, beliefs, practices, and problem-solving strategies of culturally/ethnically diverse groups"—NO, this is cultural awareness.

C. Is able to "conduct a cultural assessment in partnership with the client/ patient"—YES, this demonstrates skill.

D. Engages in "cross-cultural interactions with people who are culturally/ethnically diverse from oneself"—NO, this does not guarantee skill.

Exhibit 8-3: The Central Concepts of Campinha-Bacote (2008) Model

- *"Cultural Awareness.* The nurse becomes sensitive to the values, beliefs, lifestyle, and practices of the patient/client, and explores her/his own values, biases and prejudices. Unless the nurse goes through this process in a conscious, deliberate, and reflective manner there is always the risk of the nurse imposing her/his own cultural values during the encounter.
- *Cultural Knowledge.* Cultural knowledge is the process in which the nurse finds out more about other cultures and the different worldviews held by people from other cultures. Understanding of the values, beliefs, practices, and problem-solving strategies of culturally/ethnically diverse groups enables the nurse to gain confidence in her/his encounters with them.
- *Cultural Skill.* Cultural skill as a process is concerned with carrying out a cultural assessment. Based on the cultural knowledge gained, the nurse is able to conduct a cultural assessment in partnership with the client/patient.
- *Cultural Encounter.* Cultural encounter is the process that provides the primary and experiential exposure to cross-cultural interactions with people who are culturally/ethnically diverse from oneself.
- *Cultural Desire.* Cultural desire is an additional element to the model of cultural competence. It is seen as a self-motivational aspect of individuals and organizations to want to engage in the process of cultural competence." (American Association of Colleges of Nursing, 2008, p. 5)

Exercise 8-12: *Select all that apply*

Factors to consider in nonverbal communication include:

- ☒ **Silence**
- ☐ Socioeconomic status
- ☒ **Distance**
- ☐ Physical attributes
- ☒ **Eye contact**
- ☒ **Emotional or facial expression**
- ☐ Dietary preferences
- ☒ **Body positioning**
- ☒ **Gestures**
- ☒ **Touch**

Exercise 8-13: *Select all that apply*

The *form* of the health education material refers to:

- ☐ Concepts
- ☒ **Style**
- ☒ **Vocabulary**

☐ Perspective

☒ **Voice**

☒ **Story line**

Exercise 8-14: *True or false*

In addition, Sadie knows she must make sure that materials she develops must be readable. The *readability* of a document refers to the ease with which the eye can recognize words on a document.

  A. True

  B. False, this is legibility. Readability takes into account many factors, including the reader's skill, the text, and the language.

Exercise 8-15: *Fill-in*

Sadie realizes that health education materials must be readable. Strategies to ensure readability of patient education materials include:

  1. Use a readability tool such as SMOG/Fry to assess reading level.

  2. Develop materials at the appropriate reading level for the target audience— so one needs to assess target audience.

  3. Make written materials as clear and concise as possible.

  4. Avoid technical or health professional jargon.

  5. Avoid slang or colloquialisms.

  6. Accompany written content with good and relevant visual images. Images should "tell the story" so the reader can draw meaning from the images as well.

  7. Consider the cultural relevance of images and symbols that you are planning to use.

  8. Use font type and size that is easy to read.

Exercise 8-16: *Select all that apply*

Sadie knows that putting time into ensuring the health education materials she creates are clear, to the point, and readable will have the following benefits:

☒ **Reaches people who cannot read well or who don't have time to read well**

☐ Reduces health care costs

☒ **Helps all readers understand information**

☐ Meets the needs of all community members

☒ **Avoids misunderstandings and errors**

☒ **Avoids confusion**

☒ **Saves time (because it gets the job done well the first time)**

Exercise 8-17: *Fill-in*

Select a patient education document/pamphlet of your choice and use the SMOG and Fry Readability tools to conduct a readability analysis and compare results.

Good job completing the readability exercise!

Exercise 8-18: *Fill-in*

If the material is only available in hard copy, use Appendix C of *Simply Put* (http://goo.gl/L9SNf) to do the analysis. Do the two tools provide the same readability score?

You may notice that there is a difference between the reading level scores you get when using different tools. It is important to note the criterion the score is based upon. Some scores are based upon 100% comprehension (SMOG, ATOS), while others are based upon 75% comprehension (Fry and others).

Exercise 8-19: *Fill-in*

What is the definition of a "community"?

Community can be defined in many ways. It can be:

- **a unified body of individuals**
- **the people with common interests living in a particular area**
- **the geographic area itself**
- **an interacting population of various kinds of individuals (as species) in a common location**
- **a group of people with a common characteristic or interest living together within a larger society (a community of retired persons)**
- **a group linked by a common policy**
- **a body of persons or nations having a common history or common social, economic, and political interests (the international community)**
- **a body of persons of common and especially professional interests scattered through a larger society (e.g. the academic community) (Merriam-Webster.com, 2012)**

Exercise 8-20: *Multiple-choice question*

A windshield survey is all of the following except:

A. A composite of subjective and objective data that help define a community—NO, it does define the community.

B. Contains information about trends, stability, and changes that will affect the health of the population—NO, it is does look at all this information.

C. **Is always conducted while the observer sits in a car—YES, the nurse does not have to be in the car.**

D. Provides a visual overview of a community. A person can also perform a windshield survey by walking through the targeted area—NO, it does provide a visual overview.

E. Relies on observations for data and other information instead of directing questions to participants—NO, it does ask questions of community inhabitants.

Exercise 8-21: *Fill-in*

List the components of a windshield survey.

Exhibit 8-4: Components of a Windshield Survey

1. **Boundaries**—map or geographical structures

2. **Housing, Industry, and Zoning**

3. **Environmental Hazards and Sanitation**

4. **Open Space**—parks, empty lots, razed housing, and so forth

5. **"Commons"**—community gathering places; hangouts, are these members only?

6. **Transportation**—public, private, availability?, condition and type

7. **Service Centers**—health care, social agencies, recreation centers/facilities, hospitals, clinics, shelters

8. **Schools or Day Care**

9. **Stores**

10. **Nutritional Resources**—grocery stores, food co-ops, street vendors, food cupboards or banks, farmer's market, restaurants

11. **People on the Street**—who is out and about?

12. **Signs of Decay**

13. **Race/Ethnicity/Culture**

14. **Religion**—churches, religious organizations

15. **Safety**—police/fire stations/ambulances

16. **Politics/Policy/Political Activism**—political signs/posters, city council office, etc?

17. **Art and Cultural Centers**—museums, theater, public art

18. **Mass Media**—TV antennas, satellite dishes, other evidence of media?

Exercise 8-22: *Fill-in*

Primary data and secondary data sources include items listed in Exhibit 8-5.

Exhibit 8-5: Community Assessment Data Sources

Primary Data Collection Techniques—data directly from a client or target population

1. General survey of the population

2. Survey of a subpopulation (purposeful or stratified survey)

3. Survey of key informants (one form of a purposeful survey)

(continued)

Exhibit 8-5: Community Assessment Data Sources (*continued*)

- Includes respondents from client groups, service providers, community leaders, and so forth
- Informants by virtue of their formal community role, includes town clerks, elected officials, fire persons, mail persons, historians and librarians, all people at "nodes" of formal or "official" information exchange
- Informants by virtue of their community economic role include farmers, bartenders, general storekeepers, marina operators, all people at "nodes" of economic information exchange
- Informants by virtue of their informal roles in the community include gossips, members of various formal and informal clubs and groups, town characters, secretaries, and so on. All these have a vantage point because of their informal organizational activities

4. Observations including situations where the researcher is "known" or "unknown," as well as those where the researcher participates or doesn't participate

Secondary Data Collection Techniques—data from once collected sources

1. Some general, national level, and "public" sources:
   - U.S. Census of Housing and Population, Agriculture, Business data including the County Business Patterns and Standard Industrial Code information
   - Vital statistics
   - Service district statistics including basic client counts, attributes, demographics, social conditions, and lots of program information (analogous to public schools and schoolteachers, who constitute some of the most accountable of public servants)
   - Other social and economic indicators, Consumer Price Index, unemployment figures, inflation indicators, income figures, and so forth
   - Resource inventories and other needs assessments
   - Opinion polls taken by others
   - Budgets

2. Unusual, but easily accessible community data sources
   - State tourist maps and other state road maps
   - Topographic maps and aerial photos
   - The Yellow Pages
   - Newspapers
   - Bulletin boards
   - Films, postcards, old prints, and so forth
   - High school yearbooks and similar memorabilia

Source: Adapted from University of Vermont (1997).

Exercise 8-23: *Multiple-choice question*

Conducting interviews is considered:

A. Rapport building—NO, this is just a piece of the interview.

B. Culturally sensitive—NO, this should be but may not be the case.

C. **Primary data collection—YES, the purpose of the interview is to gain information.**

D. Secondary data collection—NO, it is primary.

Exercise 8-24: *Fill-in*

What are the overarching goals of Healthy People 2020?

Overarching goals of Healthy People 2020 include:

- **Attain high-quality, longer lives free of preventable disease, disability, injury, and premature death**
- **Achieve health equity, eliminate disparities, and improve the health of all groups**
- **Create social and physical environments that promote good health for all**
- **Promote quality of life, healthy development, and healthy behaviors across all life stages**

Exercise 8-25: *Fill-in*

What is health disparity?

If a health outcome is seen to a greater or lesser extent between populations, there is disparity. Healthy People 2020 defines a *health disparity* as "a particular type of health difference that is closely linked with social, economic, and/or environmental disadvantage. Health disparities adversely affect groups of people who have systematically experienced greater obstacles to health based on their racial or ethnic group; religion; socioeconomic status; gender; age; mental health; cognitive, sensory, or physical disability; sexual orientation or gender identity; geographic location; or other characteristics historically linked to discrimination or exclusion" (U.S. Department of Health and Human Services, 2008, p. 28). Please see Figure 8-3 for a visual representation of Healthy People 2020's overarching goals in relation to health disparities.

Figure 8-3: Action Model to Achieve Healthy People 2020 Overarching Goals

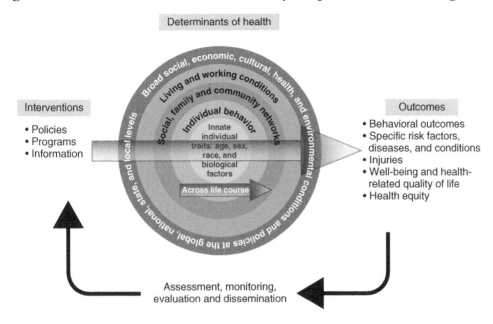

Source: U.S. Department of Health and Human Services. Phase I Report—Recommendations for the Framework and Format of Healthy People 2020. Available at: http://healthypeople. gov/2020/about/advisory/Reports.aspx

Exercise 8-26: *Multiple-choice question*

When Sadie plans culturally appropriate health education programs for the community, which of the following strategies should she use?

A. Set goals that reflect mainstream values—NO, this is not culturally sensitive.

B. Consult with local groups, leaders, and individuals—YES, this will assess the needs.

C. Use all available communication methods to get the message out—NO, this will be costly.

D. Consider using health care experts to deliver the message—NO, individuals from within the community will be responded to more favorably.

Exhibit 8-6: Answer Details

In addition to consulting with local groups, leaders, and individuals, Sadie should also:

- Set culturally acceptable goals
- Use acceptable methods of message delivery
- Consider using "in-group" members to deliver the message.

Exercise 8-27: *True or false*

For the most part, individuals have direct control over all their health determinants and can take steps to improve their own health.

A. True

B. False

Exhibit 8-7: Answer Details

It is the context of people's lives that determines their health. So it is unlikely that an individual is able to directly control all their health determinants. There are many factors that influence and frequently determine an individual's or a population's health that are beyond an individual's control.

Exercise 8-28: *Select all that apply*

Determinants of health are:

☒ **The economic factors impacting individuals or populations**

☒ **The physical environment impacting individuals or populations**

☒ **A person's individual characteristics and behaviors**

☒ **A person's genetic makeup**

☒ **The social factors impacting individuals or populations**

Exhibit 8-8: Answer Details

Determinants of health encompass a wide range of personal, social, economic, and environmental factors that impact the health status of individuals or populations.

- Social environment
- Economic environment
- Physical environment
- A person's individual characteristics and behaviors
- Income and social status
- Education
- Social support networks
- Genetics
- Health services
- Gender

For additional information, visit the following two Healthy People 2020 webpages: Disparities (http://goo.gl/CwyUJ) and Social Determinants of Health (http://goo.gl/JLWhj)

Exercise 8-29: *Fill-in*

What measures were put into place to help impact Carla's health determinants?

Measures put into place to impact Carla's determinants of health included: Keeping school gym open after school and during the summer vacation to address the determinants of health influenced by the following factors:

- **No parks or playgrounds**
- **Watches 4 hours of TV every day**
- **Lives in older building → exposure to mold and lead dust**

This change can have an impact upon health behaviors and health outcomes.

Exercise 8-30: *Matching*

Match the Model in Column A with the correct description in Column B.

Column A	Column B
A. PRECEDE-PROCEED Model	__D__ Serves as a data collection tool and planning resource for community members who want to make their community a healthier one
B. PATCH Model	__C__ Incorporates systems thinking that involves examining the underlying structure of community health issues and systems in order to create lasting positive change on a community level
C. MAPP	__A__ Premise is that a change process should focus initially on the outcome, not on the activity; it is a participatory process involving those affected by the issue or condition
D. CHANGE	__B__ Process that many communities use to collect and use local data, set health priorities, plan, conduct, and evaluate health promotion and disease prevention programs

9

Home Health Care

Unfolding Case Study #1 ▰ Seymour Jones

Mr. Jones is a 69-year-old who was discharged from the hospital yesterday following a short hospitalization to treat a leg ulcer that became increasingly worse (increased pain and inflammation) over a 2-week period prior to admission. In addition, he has a diagnosis of congestive heart failure (CHF) and diabetes. Mr. Jones lives alone in a senior citizens' high-rise.

Donna Atkins, BSN, RN, is the home care nurse assigned to visit Mr. Jones. She prepares to make this initial home visit.

Exercise 9-1: *Fill-in*
What steps should Donna take to prepare for the initial home visit?

_____

_____

_____

As Donna reviews the Continuing Patient Care Form received from the discharge planner at the hospital, she notes the following:

- 67-year-old male
- Admitted to hospital with 2-week history of infection; right leg ulcer with progressive pain
- Treatment with intravenous antibiotics
- History of CHF with shortness of breath (SOB) for 10 years
- History of diabetes for 10 years
- Home oxygen

Exercise 9-2: *Fill-in*
What is the top priority for the home care nurse during this initial home visit?

_____

_____

_____

_____

_____

Exercise 9-3: *Fill-in*
An important role for the home care nurse is that of patient or family education. Review the Continuing Patient Care referral form (Figures 9-1 and 9-2). What patient education materials should Donna consider bringing with her for this initial home visit?

_____

_____

_____

_____

Donna arrives at Mr. Jones' apartment at 10:30 a.m. She introduces herself and explains the purpose of this home visit. "Mr. Jones, your doctor has made this referral to provide you some additional support and care during the transition from the hospital to the home. He has given specific instructions for your care so that you can recover." Mr. Jones expresses concern regarding the cost of the service. "I am on a fixed income, you know, and I can't afford to pay for any service." Donna reviews the Continuing Patient Care referral form again before responding.

Exercise 9-4: *Select all that apply*
What would be correct responses to Mr. Jones?

    ❑ "Home health care services are provided free to all seniors living in the community."

    ❑ "You will have to pay a small amount of money for this service. Medicare requires that you are charged $5 co-pay for each home visit."

    ❑ "You won't need to pay anything out of pocket because you need intermittent skilled nursing care."

    ❑ "You won't need to pay anything out of pocket because you meet the criterion of being 'homebound.'"

    ❑ "You are eligible to receive home health care services because you have an order for occupational therapy."

Answers to this chapter begin on page 234.

eResource 9-1: To provide additional information regarding home care benefits under Medicare, Donna provides Mr. Jones with the following pamphlet, *Medicare and Home Health Care*: http://goo.gl/qJbuW

Figure 9-1: Continuing Patient Care Form

Patient Last Name First Name *Jones, Seymour*	**TO: CENTRAL HOME HEALTH CARE, INC.** 20245 Arbod Rd, Ste. 100 Summerville, MN (555) 555-5410 Fax: (555) 555-5412	
Address for Care City or Twp *700 Shadyside Manor Drive, Apt 804, Summerville, MN* Phone (555) 555-1234	FROM: Hospital, Clinic, E.C.F. and Address Grand Valley Medical Center	
Patient's Address, if not same as above Phone	Referral Date: 3/16 Reported by: Agency 1ˢᵗ Visit: 3/17 Reported to: Date:	
Complete Birth Date Sex Marital Status Ⓜ F S M Ⓦ D Sep	Hospital for Drugs or Services Grand Valley Medical Center	
Responsible Relative or Friend	Medicare No. 099-44-4444	
	Medicaid No	
Relationship Phone	Blue Cross No.	
Hospital Case No. Room No. Admission 3/8 Discharge 3/16	Other Ins. (Give Name) Aetna policy #223230234	

II REPORT BY PHYSICIAN

Diagnosis: List Primary First and Date of Onset *R leg ulcer 3/8* *CHF x 10 years; DM x 10 years*	Prognosis Good ☒ Fair ☐ Guarded ☐ Poor ☐ Patient Informed of Diagnosis Yes ☒ No ☐ Family Informed of Diagnosis Yes ☒ No ☐
Surgery Performed (Type and Date): *N/A* Complications: none	Brief Medical History: *Adm to hosp with 2 wk hx of infection; R leg ulcer with* *progressive pain; TX with IV Antibiotics* *Hx of CHF with SOB* *Hx of Diabetes*
Rehabilitation or Treatment Goal: *Wound healing, Stable CHF* *and Diabetes*	Date and Place of Physician's Next Visit: 2 weeks Home ☐ Office ☒ Clinic ☐ E.C.F. ☐

MEDICAL ORDERS AND PLAN OF TREATMENT

Diet (Specify) *1800 ADA* Dressing or Treatment (Specify) *Dry dressing R leg ulcer BID, Cleanse with NS, pat dry, apply dry dsg (clean technique)*	Minimum Number of Hosp. Days Saved ☐

Catheter ☐ Size _____ Frequency Change _____ Irrigation Solution _____ Amount _____ Frequency _____
Enema (Specify)
Medications:
- *Prandin 3.5 mg po before meals*
- *Lasix 40 mg qd (New medication)*
- *Keflex 500 mg 2 tabs (1gm total) po q6 hours x 7d*

Specify Therapeutic Exercise Program

Activity Allowance:
    As tolerated
Patient Uses: Prostheses ☐   Brace ☐   Walker ☒   Wheelchair ☐   Cane ☐   Other _____
Physical Therapy ☒ Occupational Therapy ☒   Social Service ☐   Speech ☐   Evaluate Need for Home Health Aide ☒

Teaching Patient or Family:

I certify that the above patient is under my care and requires the above Home Health Service because he is confined to his home. These professional services are to be provided on an intermittent basis and the established plan contained in the record will be reviewed by me at least every two months. These services are needed to treat all of the conditions for which the patient was treated during the related in-patient hospital or post-hospital extended care facility approved stay.

Date 3/25 Physician's Signature *Dr. smith* Address Grand Valley Med Ctr   Phone (555) 555-3333   Signed by Resident

She also notes on the back of the referral form the following:

Figure 9-2: Continuing Patient Care Form

III. HOSPITAL NURSE'S ASSESSMENT: Reason for Referral?

Activity Limitations:
Ambulatory ☐
Ambulatory with Assistance ☒
Confined to Bed ☐ Chair ☐

Mental State:
Alert ☒   Depressed ☒
Apathetic ☐   Disoriented ☐
Confused ☐   Other _____
　　　　Upset re: decreased mobility

Disabilities and Impairments:
Mentality ☐
Speech ☐
Hearing ☐
Vision ☒ - glasses
Sensation ☒ - diabetic
Neuropathy ☐
Amputation ☐
Paralysis ☐
Contractures ☐
Decubiti ☐

Allergies: NKA
Special Problems and Other Narrative:
　　O$_2$ at 2LPM per nasal cannula

Activities of Daily Living:
Independent ☐
Needs Assistance ☒
Unable to do ☐

Incontinence:

	None	Partial	Complete
Bowel	☒	☐	☐
Bladder	☒	☐	☐

In-Hospital Teaching:
Bowel Training _____
Bladder Training _____
Colostomy Care _____
Insulin Administration _____
Modified Diet Instructions ☐
Copy of Diet to Patient ☒
Copy of Diet to Agency ☒
Other _____
Other Significant Finding:

Vital Signs with Ranges & Dates:
TPR 99.8 – 90.28
BP 136/90
WT 165.0
Weight daily, call Dr. Smith if wt gain >2 lbs in 24 hours or >5 lbs in 7 days.

X-Ray: Findings & Dates:

Laboratory: Findings & Dates:
Hb. B.S. 7.3% - 3/15

BUN 8.4mg/dL – 3/9

Culture Serology

After washing her hands, Donna begins the initial assessment, taking vital signs and reviewing the discharge materials provided to the patient upon discharge from the hospital. Mr. Jones' vital signs are: BP—140/88, T—99.2°, AR—90, RR—32. He has a soiled dressing on his R lower leg. Bilateral edema: Right leg is more edematous than the left: R leg — +3 pitting; L leg — +2 pitting.

Mr. Jones denies any chest pain but does report being short of breath more than before the hospitalization. He complains that he fatigues more easily. He uses two pillows at night in order to breathe comfortably. Mr. Jones reports an occasional cough that sometimes raises some frothy white sputum.

Donna notices a chart for recording daily weights and asks the patient if he has weighed himself today. He replies "No, I figured you would do it when you came."

Donna looks around the room and notices that Mr. Jones' walker is across the room. She brings the walker within his reach and observes his ability to get up and ambulate. Donna observes that Mr. Jones is able to ambulate slowly using a walker but appears to get shortness of breath with minimal exertion. Mr. Jones expresses frustration regarding his decreased ability to ambulate. She provides encouragement.

Answers to this chapter begin on page 234.

Exercise 9-5: *Fill-in*

What additional instruction is warranted for Mr. Jones regarding safe ambulation and managing activities with CHF?

_____

_____

_____

_____

Mr. Jones ambulates to the bathroom where the digital scale is located. Donna makes sure that the scale is functioning properly and stands close to Mr. Jones as he stands on the scale. Mr. Jones' weight is 166.1. Donna documents the weight on the chart and compares it with the weight recorded on the continuing patient care form.

Figure 9-3

Date	Weight
3/16	165.0
3/17	166.1
3/18	
3/19	
3/20	
3/21	
3/22	

Exercise 9-6: *Multiple-choice question*

Donna notices that Mr. Jones' weight is higher than it was in the hospital yesterday. Mr. Jones asks, "Is that a bad thing?" What is the best response for Donna to give?

    A. This is nothing to worry about, but it is something we should monitor.

    B. We need to call your doctor. He will want to adjust your medication.

    C. This is something that we need to monitor closely because weight gain can be an early signal that you are retaining fluid.

    D. Have you been eating foods high in salt? That can be the cause of your weight gain.

Exercise 9-7: *Fill-in*

What specific instructions should Donna provide to Mr. Jones?

_____

_____

_____

_____

Answers to this chapter begin on page 234.

Donna asks Mr. Jones about his diabetes and how he has been managing it. He shows her his Blood Sugar Record. "I've been a diabetic for more than 10 years now and have been managing that pretty well. This leg thing is what messed me up. I just don't understand why. I have been doing everything the same as always and taking my sugar pill."

Figure 9-4

Date	Morning BS	Evening BS	Comments
3/15	100	140	
3/16	110	160	
3/17	98	134	
3/18	120		
3/19			
3/20			
3/21			
3/22			

Exercise 9-8: *Multiple-choice question*

What would be the best response for Donna to give to Mr. Jones?

A. "You must have eaten something that you shouldn't have and that's what has thrown off your blood sugar levels."

B. "Diabetes affects how your body responds to infection. It was good that you went to the doctor when you started having problems with your leg."

C. "When your body is fighting an infection, it is important to increase your dietary calories to provide nutrients for healing."

D. "When your body has an infection, it really doesn't matter what you do, you just have to let it run its course."

Donna reviews the Blood Sugar Record and asks Mr. Jones to show her how he checks his blood sugar. He pulls out his glucometer and very proficiently demonstrates how he performs a blood sugar test. Donna asks Mr. Jones about his diabetes medication. He reports he takes it as directed without fail.

 eResource 9-2: Donna refers to the drug guide, Epocrates, to review the common side effects and potential adverse reactions to this medication: [Pathway: https://online.epocrates.com → select "Drugs" tab → enter "Prandin" into the search field → select "Adverse Reactions"]

Donna asks Mr. Jones about his diet. "Well, I was always on a 1,800 calorie diet . . . from the beginning when I was first diagnosed. I know that I am supposed to use a different method but I am a little fuzzy on that new method." Donna tells Mr. Jones, "The new method focuses on portion sizes so it makes it easier to eat healthy."

 eResource 9-3: To reinforce the instruction she provided, Donna shows Mr. Jones a brief video tutorial from the American Diabetes Association, *Diabetes Basics: Create Your Plate:* http://youtu.be/A6LZijdsGu0

Answers to this chapter begin on page 234.

Following the video, Donna asks Mr. Jones to do a 24-hour dietary recall.

Exhibit 9-1: 24-Hour Dietary Recall

- Breakfast yesterday (at the hospital): Two scrambled eggs, two slices of toast with butter and jelly, coffee, and orange juice
- Lunch (at home): Canned tomato soup with crackers and grilled cheese sandwich
- Dinner: Stouffer's Chicken Pot Pie, coleslaw, and a glass of 2% milk
- Breakfast today: Oatmeal, coffee, and a banana

Exercise 9-9: *Fill-in*

What additional dietary teaching should Donna provide to Mr. Jones?

_____

_____

_____

Mr. Jones reports that he tests his blood sugar twice a day. He denies being excessively thirsty. "I think it seems like I am going to the bathroom more than before I was in the hospital; maybe it just seems that way because I get tired so easily."

Donna reviews the medications on the Continuing Patient Care form and verifies the labels on the prescription bottles.

Mr. Jones' medications are:

- Prandin 3.5 mg orally before meals
- Lasix 40 mg orally every day (new medication)
- Keflex 500 mg—two tabs (1 g total) orally every 6 hours for 7 days

Exercise 9-10: *Fill-in*

What additional medication teaching does Mr. Jones need at this time?

_____

_____

_____

 eResource 9-4: To reinforce medication teaching she has done with additional patient education materials, Donna refers to the drug guide, Epocrates: [Pathway: https://online.epocrates.com → select "Drugs" tab → enter "Lasix" into the search field → select "Patient Education"]

Answers to this chapter begin on page 234.

Donna continues the home visit and learns the following about Mr. Jones:

- He has been widowed for the past 15 years and seems to have adjusted to single life.
- He has several friends in the building whom he can call and ask for help.
- He is highly motivated to resume his independent life, but seems afraid it will not be possible.
- His hobbies included cooking for friends, playing poker with friends.

When Donna learns that Mr. Jones enjoys cooking, she shows him the American Diabetes Association's (ADA's) website where there are some good recipes that he can try out.

eResource 9-5: To provide additional dietary and diabetic management support, including access to recipes, meal plans, tips, and other tools, she helps him sign up for ADA's My Food Advisor program: [Pathway: www .diabetes.org → select "Food and Fitness" → select "MyFoodAdvisor"]

eResource 9-6: Donna tells Mr. Jones about a variety of mobile tools to help him manage his diabetes:
Apple IOS
- Diabetes Companion by dLife, a comprehensive diabetes mobile application: http://goo.gl/MGJ6T
- Diabetes App Lite—blood sugar control, glucose tracker, and carbohydrate counter by BHI Technologies, Inc.: http://goo.gl/lXUKJ
- Glucose Buddy—Diabetes Helper 3.6.5 by Azumio Inc.: http://goo.gl/Rv6N3

Android OS
- OnTrack Diabetes by GExperts Inc.: http://goo.gl/2MeHB
- Glucool Diabetes by 3qubits http://goo.gl/Iebrn

Donna turns her attention to assess the leg wound. She washes her hands again and sets up her workspace. She positions Mr. Jones leg so that he is comfortable and she is able to safely provide care. She verifies the wound care order on the Continuing Patient Care form.

Exercise 9-11: *Fill-in*
When providing wound care, what characteristics of the wound must be assessed?

_____

_____

_____

eResource 9-7: For additional information regarding wound assessment, refer to: Clinical Wound Assessment—A Pocket Guide: http://goo.gl/0I8HM

Answers to this chapter begin on page 234.

Mr. Jones looks at his wound and asks Donna how the wound looks to her. She responds that the wound is still in the inflammatory phase of wound healing. He is puzzled and asks more questions.

 eResource 9-8: To help Mr. Jones understand the phases of wound healing, Donna shows him a brief video: http://youtu.be/u7Ryg9nVFLI

Donna completes the wound care and provides verbal and written instructions regarding caring and monitoring the wound.

Exercise 9-12: *Fill-in*
What additional instructions should Donna provide to Mr. Jones?

_____

_____

_____

Donna completes her initial home visit. She summarizes all the information she has shared and provides specific instructions in writing. Mindful that patient safety is a priority concern, she reviews the signs and symptoms (S/S) of complications that warrant immediate action and when to call the nurse or doctor. Donna provides a list of emergency phone numbers. Finally, she makes arrangements for a follow-up home visit in 2 days.

Answers to this chapter begin on page 234.

Answers

Exercise 9-1: *Fill-in*

What steps should Donna take to prepare for the initial home visit?

1. **Review the referral form, clarify information and orders if need be**

2. **Contact patient/family to arrange home visit, verify address/directions, and identify if any supplies are needed**

3. **Collect required admission paperwork**

4. **Assemble required supplies (e.g., dressing supplies, etc.)**

5. **Assemble anticipated patient education material**

6. **Plan focus of home visit (e.g., initial home visit will involve complete patient and home assessment; admission interview and paperwork; initial patient teaching; home safety, etc.)**

Exercise 9-2: *Fill-in*

What is the top priority for the home care nurse during this initial home visit?

Patient safety is the top priority for this initial home visit. Home safety and emergency information materials (this is a critical component of the first home visit and should be followed up on in subsequent home visits. The home care nurse must make sure the patient is safe, health status is stable, and either the patient or the caregiver can take appropriate action if necessary; that is, O₂ safety, S/S to report to the doctor, S/S warranting immediate transport to the emergency room).

Exercise 9-3: *Fill-in*

An important role for the home care nurse is that of patient/family education. Review the Continuing Patient Care referral form (Figures 9-1 and 9-2). What patient education materials should Donna consider bringing with her for this initial home visit?

Donna should plan on doing patient teaching on the following:

1. **Medication instruction sheets for Lasix, Prandin, and Keflix**

2. **Diabetic diet (1800 ADA)**

3. **Managing CHF**

4. **Daily weight**

5. **Wound care**

Exercise 9-4: *Select all that apply*

What would the correct response to Mr. Jones be?

❑ Home health care services are provided free to all seniors living in the community.

❑ You will have to pay a small amount of money for this service. Medicare requires that you are charged $5 co-pay for each home visit.

☒ **You won't need to pay anything out of pocket because you need intermittent skilled nursing care.**

☒ **You won't need to pay anything out of pocket because you meet the criterion of being "homebound."**

❑ You are eligible to receive home health care services because you have an order for occupational therapy.

Exhibit 9-2: Answer Details

For more information, please review: *Medicare and Home Health Care*: http://www.medicare.gov/publications/pubs/pdf/10969.pdf

Exercise 9-5: *Fill-in*

What additional instruction is warranted for Mr. Jones regarding safe ambulation and managing activities with CHF?

- **Physical therapy will help with improving your activity tolerance.**

- **It is recommended that you gradually increase your activity. It is important to avoid activities that put abrupt demands on the heart.**

- **Intersperse activities with periods of rest. Be sure to stop and rest if you feel tired or short of breath.**

- **Know your limits and do not push yourself.**

- **When in doubt, "Ask." Your doctor will be happy to give you specific instructions on how much you should exercise.**

Exercise 9.6: *Multiple-choice question*

Donna notices that Mr. Jones' weight is higher than it was in the hospital yesterday. Mr. Jones asks, "Is that a bad thing?" What is the best response for Donna to give?

A. "This is nothing to worry about but it is something we should monitor."—NO, this gives false reassurance.

B. "We need to call your doctor. He will want adjust your medication."—NO, this is not a nursing order.

C. **"This is something that we need to monitor closely because weight gain can be an early signal that you are retaining fluid."—YES, this is teaching.**

D. "Have you been eating foods high in salt? That can be the cause of your weight gain."—NO, this is accusatory.

Exercise 9-7: *Fill-in*

What specific instructions should Donna provide to Mr. Jones?

- **Daily weight—at the same time each day first thing in the morning after urinating**
- **Watch for**
  - ○ **swelling of abdomen (see how clothes fit; tightness of abdomen)**
  - ○ **increased shortness of breath or increased fatigue**
- **Call the doctor if:**
  - ○ **weight gain more than 2 lb in 24 hours or more than 5 lb in 7 days**
  - ○ **swelling of abdomen**
  - ○ **increased shortness of breath**
  - ○ **increased fatigue**

Exercise 9-8: *Multiple-choice question*

What would be the best response for Donna to give to Mr. Jones?

A. "You must have eaten something that you shouldn't have and that is what has thrown off your blood sugar levels."—NO, this is accusatory and nontherapeutic.

B. **"Diabetes affects how your body responds to infection. It was good that you went to the doctor when you started having problems with your leg."—YES, this reaffirms the patient's decision.**

C. "When your body is fighting an infection, it is important to increase your dietary calories to provide nutrients for healing."—NO, protein-poor calories do not help.

D. "When your body has an infection, it really doesn't matter what you do, you just have to let it run its course."—NO, this is dangerous advice.

Exercise 9-9: *Fill-in*

What additional dietary teaching should Donna provide to Mr. Jones?

Diet is high in sodium and fat (canned soup, chicken pot pie, grilled cheese sandwich); diet is low in vegetables.

Exercise 9-10: *Fill-in*

What additional medication teaching does Mr. Jones need at this time?

Mr. Jones has a new medication, Lasix, for which he needs instruction. Particularly, Mr. Jones needs to know the purpose, effect, and side effects of this medication.

Exercise 9-11: *Fill-in*

When providing wound care, what characteristics of the wound must be assessed?

- **Acute or chronic**
- **Type of wound (pressure, venous, arterial, surgical, tear, neuropathic/diabetic)**
- **Location**

- **Measurement of the wound**
- **Pain**
- **Edema**
- **Exudate—amount, color, consistency, and odor**
- **Wound edge/margin**
- **Surrounding skin temperature and appearance**
- **Wound bed appearance**
- **Signs and symptoms of infection**

For more information, review Morgan, N. (2010). *Wound assessment: The basic's.* Wound Care Education Institute. Available: http://goo.gl/uWS9f

Exercise 9-12: *Fill-in*
What additional instructions should Donna provide to Mr. Jones?
Mr. Jones should be instructed to monitor his wound for increased drainage, foul odor, increased pain, tenderness, swelling, and elevated temperature.

10

Health Education

Unfolding Case Study #1 — Health Literacy

Janice Berry is a nurse working as a health educator at the public health department in Raleigh, North Carolina. Her role is to conduct health education classes for the community. She conducts general health education programs—often at the request of various community groups—and a series of focused education programs designed for specific groups such as diabetics and asthmatics.

Janice knows that adults approach learning differently than children. Therefore, when developing and delivering educational programs, Janice keeps the Knowles' principles of adult learning in mind.

Exercise 10-1: *Fill-in*
What are the Knowles' principles of adult learning?

1. _____

2. _____

3. _____

4. _____

5. _____

6. _____

Exercise 10-2: *Select all that apply*
Knowles' theory of adult learning makes several assumptions about adult learners. Which of the following statements are correct?

- ❑ Adult learners need to know why they need to learn something before undertaking to learn it.
- ❑ Adults need to be responsible for their own decisions and to be treated as capable of self-direction.
- ❑ Adult learners have a more difficult time with affective learning than their younger counterparts.

Answers to this chapter begin on page 248.

❏ Adult learners have a variety of experiences of life that represent the richest resource for learning. These experiences are, however, instilled with bias and presupposition.

❏ Adult learners rely more heavily on written and visual materials when acquiring new knowledge and skills.

❏ Adult learners are ready to learn those things they need to know in order to cope effectively with life situations.

❏ Adults are motivated to learn to the extent that they perceive that it will help them perform tasks they confront in their life situations (Queensland Occupational Therapy Fieldwork Collaborative [QOTFC], 2007).

Exercise 10-3: *Fill-in*
What are the three domains of learning?

1. _____

2. _____

3. _____

Exercise 10-4: *Fill-in*
Provide examples of activities that would be used in each of the three learning domains.

Table 10-1

Domain	Learning Activity Example

Janice knows that the three primary learning styles are: visual, auditory, and kinesthetic.

Exercise 10-5: *Multiple-choice question*
Kinesthetic learners learn best by

        A. Reading text out loud and using a tape recorder

        B. Sitting at the front of the classroom to avoid visual distractions

        C. A hands-on approach and actively exploring the physical world around them

        D. Taking detailed notes to absorb information

Answers to this chapter begin on page 248.

Janice prepares learning activities using all three styles because she knows that the research has shown that learners retain approximately 10% of what they *see*; 30% to 40% of what they *see and hear*; and 90% of what we *see, hear, and do* (National Highway Institute, n.d., p. 2).

Exercise 10-6: *True or false*
Learners have the capability to use all three learning styles with equal effect.

    A. True

    B. False

 eResource 10-1: Janice uses the following virtual resources to support effective teaching:
- Centers for Disease Control's *Simply Put: A Guide for Creating Easy-to-Understand Materials*: http://goo.gl/L9SNf
- *The Clinical Educator's Toolkit*: www.qotfc.edu.au/resource
- *Quick Guide to Health Literacy*: http://goo.gl/Inr7m; and the Health Literacy Universal Precautions Toolkit: http://goo.gl/K6NXe

Janice is aware that literacy and health literacy are a problem in the community she serves. She and her colleagues are acutely aware that low literacy and low health literacy have a negative impact upon the health of the community (DeWalt et al, 2010).

Exercise 10-7: *Fill-in*
What is literacy?

_____

_____

In reviewing the literature, Janice has learned that there are three types of literacy. These include:

1. "Prose literacy: The knowledge and skills needed to perform prose tasks (i.e., to search, comprehend, and use continuous texts). Examples include editorials, news stories, brochures, and instructional materials.

2. Document literacy: The knowledge and skills needed to perform document tasks (i.e., to search, comprehend, and use noncontinuous texts in various formats). Examples include job applications, payroll forms, transportation schedules, maps, tables, and drug or food labels.

3. Quantitative literacy: The knowledge and skills required to perform quantitative tasks (i.e., to identify and perform computations, either alone or sequentially, using numbers embedded in printed materials). Examples include balancing a checkbook, figuring out a tip, completing an order form or determining the amount" (Institute of Education Sciences National Center for Education Statistics, 2003).

Answers to this chapter begin on page 248.

Exercise 10-8: *True or false*

For health literacy, only prose and document literacy are important because individuals need to be able to read and understand health information.

    A. True

    B. False

Exercise 10-9: *Fill-in*

What is health literacy?

_____

_____

 eResource 10-2: To supplement her understanding of the problem of health literacy, Janice views two videos:

    ■ The American Medical Association's video *Health Literacy and Patient Safety: Help Patients Understand*: http://youtu.be/cGtTZ_vxjyA

    ■ American Colleges of Physicians' *Health Literacy Video*: http://goo.gl/qA9BK

Janice knows that health literacy is dependent on individual and systemic factors, which include factors such as the communication skills of both the individual and the health care provider. She knows that other factors should also be considered.

Exercise 10-10: *Multiple-choice question*

Health literacy is dependent on individual and systemic factors, which include all of the following except:

    A. Genetics

    B. Culture

    C. Context

    D. Knowledge

Exercise 10-11: *Fill-in*

The consequences of poor health literacy include:

    1. _____

    2. _____

    3. _____

    4. _____

    5. _____

    6. _____

Janice and her colleagues periodically review and prepare educational materials for the populations they serve. All materials are reviewed for readability using a SMOG or Fry Formula to make sure the materials are at the proper reading level.

Answers to this chapter begin on page 248.

eResource 10-3: To help guide their work on this project, the group uses
■ North Carolina's Health Literacy Program on Health Literacy as a guide: http://nchealthliteracy.org
■ Office of Disease Prevention and Health Promotion's Health Literacy Online: http://goo.gl/yi331

Exercise 10-12: *Multiple-choice question*

Health education material should be written at a(n):

    A. Second grade reading level

    B. Third to fifth grade reading level

    C. Fifth to seventh grade reading level

    D. Eighth to ninth grade reading level

 eResource 10-4: Janice reviews the Agency for Healthcare Research and Quality's Health Literacy Universal Precautions Toolkit as she continues to prepare health education materials: http://goo.gl/LBoRC

While Janice was preparing health information handouts about a variety of commonly seen health concerns, her colleague Samantha stops by to take a look. Samantha notices that Janice has included medical terminology in the materials. She points out to her that these terms might be confusing to individuals with low health literacy. "Why not substitute these words for something simpler?" Samantha shows Janice a few examples. "I think it is important to make sure we avoid health care jargon when preparing the materials, don't you?"

Table 10-2

Medical Jargon and Simpler Alternatives	
Instead of using these terms . . .	Try using these simpler words
Jaundice	Yellow
Immunization	Shots
Myocardial infarction	Heart attack
Conjunctivitis	Pink eye
Hypertension	High blood pressure
Otitis media	Earache

Source: Mayer and Villaire (2009).

 eResource 10-5: Samantha shares a web-based *Plain Language Thesaurus* that lists plain language alternatives for medical terms: www.mmc.org/Thesaurus

Samantha tells Janice that another strategy to help improve clarity of health education materials is to use an *active voice* when giving instructions.

Answers to this chapter begin on page 248.

Exercise 10-13: *Multiple-choice question*

An example of active voice instructions is:

      A. This medicine should be taken with food.

      B. Your feet should be elevated.

      C. Walk 30 minutes daily.

      D. This form must be signed by you.

 eResource 10-6: Janice knows that using a strategy called "Teach Back" is very effective in health education. To review this method prior to using it with her next client, she watches a video demonstrating this approach: http://youtu.be/IKxjmpD7vfY

Unfolding Case Study #2   Community Education

As part of National Bike Month, Janice was invited to do a presentation on bike safety at a local elementary school. The school nurse, Lisa Kennedy, tells Janice that as part of the school program to get students to be fit, they are encouraging students to ride their bikes to school; therefore, a program on bike safety is needed. Lisa is using National Bike Month as a platform to launch a physical activity program. Lisa knows that in order to have a successful program, it is important to partner with other organizations and key stakeholders.

Exercise 10-14: *Fill-in*

Potential partners and key stakeholders that Lisa should seek out include:

_____

_____

_____

_____

Exercise 10-15: *Multiple-choice question*

A bike safety presentation is

      A. Primary prevention

      B. Secondary prevention

      C. Tertiary prevention

      D. Proactive prevention

Answers to this chapter begin on page 248.

Exercise 10-16: *Multiple-choice question*
Janice is glad to be invited to do the bike safety presentation because she knows that unintentional injuries such as those that can occur while biking are the:

    A. Leading cause of death among children
    B. Leading cause of death among young adults
    C. Leading cause of death across all age groups
    D. A and B

Janice reminds herself that for the health education program to be effective, she needs to be attentive to the needs of both adults and children. She also knows that she needs to consider the cognitive, affective, and kinesthetic domains.

Exercise 10-17: *Multiple-choice question*
Which of the following activities would best target the cognitive domain to ensure that parents understand the new bicycle helmet program?

    A. Watching a movie about bicycle maintenance
    B. A lecture and film about helmet use
    C. Role playing activities
    D. Hands-on practice with a variety of helmets

Exercise 10-18: *Multiple-choice question*
At the presentation, Janice provides information about the incidence of injury, the likelihood of injury, the severity of injury, as well as the simple steps that can be taken to protect health. Using this approach, she is applying which of the following?

    A. Stages of Change Model
    B. Transtheoretical Model
    C. Health Belief Model
    D. Self-Efficacy Model

 eResource 10-7: Janice shows the students and parents two videos:
    ▪ *Ride Smart—It's Time to Start:* http://goo.gl/wpP3I
    ▪ *Bike Safe—Bike Smart:* http://goo.gl/DH23n

The videos generate good discussion among attendees, particularly in relation to the risk of head injuries. Lisa uses this opportunity to teach about concussions—a mild form of traumatic brain injury (TBI)—because she knows that head injuries, whether from a bicycle accident or a fall on the playground, are a concern for school-age children. Lisa knows that an estimated 1.7 million people sustain a TBI annually and that about 75% of TBIs that occur each year are concussions or other forms of mild TBI (CDC, 2003; Faul, Xu, Wald, & Coronado, 2010).

 eResource 10-8: Lisa tells the attendees about the ABC's of Concussion Campaign:
    ▪ Fact Sheet: http://goo.gl/LB5oG
    ▪ Checklist: http://goo.gl/L2ejB

Answers to this chapter begin on page 248.

Exercise 10-19: *Multiple-choice question*
Providing this information to parents and teachers is
    A. Primary prevention
    B. Secondary prevention
    C. Tertiary prevention
    D. Health protection

Exercise 10-20: *Multiple-choice question*
When Lisa uses the checklist to assess a child who has fallen off the monkey bars, she is engaging in:
    A. Primary prevention
    B. Secondary prevention
    C. Tertiary prevention
    D. Health protection

Exercise 10-21: *True or false*
A person who has had a concussion would show external evidence of a head injury such as a cut, bruise, or bump.
    A. True
    B. False

Janice and Lisa realize that for any change to take place there needs to be a planned and structured approach. They realize that it is essential that the educator have an understanding of the multitude of factors that affect/influence behavior.

Lisa recalls that models and theories can help the nurse understand what influences behavior and this understanding can help in the design of effective health education programs. These theories can be organized in three broad categories: (a) Individual (Intrapersonal) Health Behavior Models/Theories, (b) Interpersonal Health Behavior Theories, and (c) Community Level Models/Theories (Campbell, 2001).

 eResource 10-9: To learn more about theoretical models related to community health education and health promotion activities, Lisa reviews: http://goo.gl/az1ZO

Exercise 10-22: *Multiple-choice question*
A model that focuses on health promotion from an interpersonal level is:
    A. The Health Belief Model
    B. The Theory of Reasoned Action
    C. The Ecological Model
    D. Stages of Change

Answers to this chapter begin on page 248.

Exercise 10-23: *Multiple-choice question*

The perspective that an individual progresses through five levels related to readiness to change—precontemplation, contemplation, preparation, action, and maintenance—when adopting new health behaviors is part of which theory?

    A. The Health Belief Model

    B. The Theory of Reasoned Action

    C. The Ecological Model

    D. Stages of Change

Exercise 10-24: *Multiple-choice question*

When Janice considers multiple levels of influence such as intrapersonal, interpersonal, institutional, community, and public policy when planning her health promotion program, she is using which of the following?

    A. The Health Belief Model

    B. The Theory of Reasoned Action

    C. The Ecological Model

    D. Stages of Change

Answers to this chapter begin on page 248.

Answers

Exercise 10-1: *Fill-in*

What are the Knowles' principles of adult learning?

Knowles identified the six principles of adult learning outlined below.
1. "Adults are internally motivated and self-directed."
2. "Adults bring life experiences and knowledge to learning experiences."
3. "Adults are goal oriented."
4. "Adults are relevancy oriented."
5. "Adults are practical."
6. "Adult learners like to be respected (Atherton, 2011, p. 2)."

Exercise 10-2: *Select all that apply*

Knowles' theory of adult learning makes several assumptions about adult learners. Which of the following statements are correct?

☒ **Adult learners need to know why they need to learn something before undertaking to learn it.**

☒ **Adults need to be responsible for their own decisions and to be treated as capable of self-direction.**

☐ Adult learners have a more difficult time with affective learning than their younger counterparts.

☒ **Adult learners have a variety of experiences of life that represent the richest resource for learning. These experiences are, however, instilled with bias and presupposition.**

☐ Adult learners rely more heavily on written and visual materials when acquiring new knowledge and skills.

☒ **Adult learners are ready to learn those things they need to know in order to cope effectively with life situations.**

☒ **Adults are motivated to learn to the extent that they perceive that it will help them perform tasks they confront in their life situations (QOTFC, 2007).**

Exercise 10-3: *Fill-in*

What are the three domains of learning?
1. Cognitive
2. Affective
3. Behavioral (psychomotor)

Exercise 10-4: *Fill-in*

Provide examples of activities that would be used in each of the three learning domains.

Table 10-3

Domain	Learning Activity Example
Cognitive	**Lecture, discussions, brainstorming activities**
Affective	**Values clarification exercises, group process activities, consensus building activities**
Behavioral	**Role playing, demonstration, teach backs, simulation**

Exercise 10-5: *Multiple-choice question*

Kinesthetic learners learn best by

A. Reading text out loud and using a tape recorder—NO, this would be best for auditory learners.

B. Sitting at the front of the classroom to avoid visual distractions—NO, this is a method for visual learners.

C. **A hands-on approach and actively exploring the physical world around them—YES**

D. Taking detailed notes to absorb information—NO, this is a method of learning for behavioral or psychomotor learners.

Exercise 10-6: *True or false*

Learners have the capability to use all three learning styles with equal effect.

A. True

B. **False**

Exhibit 10-1: Answer Details

While learners have the capability to learn via all three styles, they are usually dominant in one.

Exercise 10-7: *Fill-in*

What is literacy?

Literacy can be defined as a person's ability to read, write, speak, compute, and solve problems at levels necessary to:

- **Function on the job and in society**
- **Achieve one's goals**
- **Develop one's knowledge and potential**

Exhibit 10-2: Answer Details

The term "illiteracy" means being unable to read or write. A person who has limited or low literacy skills is not illiterate.

The National Literacy Act of 1991, Pub. L No. 102-73.

Exercise 10-8: *True or false*
For health literacy, only prose and document literacy are important because individuals need to be able to read and understand health information.
A. True
B. False

Exhibit 10-3: Answer Details

Quantitative literacy is also important in health literacy because patients need to be able to understand dosages and equivalencies. In addition, patients need to be able to measure medications (e.g., insulin, liquid medications, etc.).

Exercise 10-9: *Fill-in*
What is health literacy?
Health literacy is the degree to which individuals have the capacity to obtain, process, and understand basic health information and services needed to make appropriate health decisions (U.S. Department of Health and Human Services Office of Disease Prevention and Health Promotion [USDHHS ODPHP], October 28, 2012).

Exercise 10-10: *Multiple-choice question*
Health literacy is dependent on individual and systemic factors, which include all of the following except:
A. Genetics—YES, this is not a determinant of literacy.
B. Culture—NO, this does play a part in an individual's ability to read.
C. Context—NO, this does play a part in an individual's ability to read.
D. Knowledge—NO, this does play a part in an individual's ability to read.

Exercise 10-11: *Fill-in*
The consequences of poor health literacy include:
 Individuals with low health literacy are:

 1. **Less likely to use preventive health care services (mammograms, Pap smears, flu shots, etc.)**

 2. **Have less knowledge about medical conditions and treatment and therefore are more likely to have chronic conditions and be less able to manage these effectively**

 3. **Have increased hospitalizations and increased use of the emergency department**

 4. **More likely to have poor health status**

5. **Have higher health care costs because of deferred health care, less use of preventive services resulting in requiring more costly health care**

6. **More likely to have negative psychological effects associated with a sense of shame and being stigmatized due to limited health literacy skills (USDHHS ODPHP, October 28, 2012)**

Exercise 10-12: *Multiple-choice question*
Health education material should be written at a(n):
A. Second grade reading level—NO, this is too low a level.
B. Third to fifth grade reading level—YES
C. Fifth to seventh grade reading level—NO, this may be too high a level for some.
D. Eighth to ninth grade reading level—NO, too high a level.

Exercise 10-13: *Multiple-choice question*
An example of active voice instructions is:
A. This medicine should be taken with food—NO, this is passive.
B. Your feet should be elevated—NO, this is also passive.
C. Walk 30 minutes daily—YES, this is active and direct.
D. This form must be signed by you—NO, this is also passive tense.

Exercise 10-14: *Fill-in*
Potential partners and key stakeholders that Lisa should seek out include:
- **bike clubs and coalitions**
- **bike shops**
- **chambers of commerce**
- **other schools**
- **community centers**
- **restaurants**
- **museums**
- **local businesses and employers**
- **churches**
- **health care providers**

Exercise 10-15: *Multiple-choice question*
A bike safety presentation is
A. Primary prevention—YES, this is teaching people to be safe before any incident happens.
B. Secondary prevention—NO, this is screening.
C. Tertiary prevention—NO, this is interventional after an incident happens.
D. Proactive prevention—NO, this term is not used.

Exercise 10-16: *Multiple-choice question*

Janice is glad to be invited to do the bike safety presentation because she knows that unintentional injuries such as those that can occur while biking are the:

A. Leading cause of death among children—YES

B. Leading cause of death among young adults—YES

C. Leading cause of death across all age groups—NO, in later years it is other causes.

D. A and B

Exhibit 10-4: Answer Details

Each year, more than 500,000 people in the United States are treated in emergency departments, and more than 700 people die as a result of bicycle-related injuries. Children are at particularly high risk for bicycle-related injuries. In 2001, children 15 years and younger accounted for 59% of all bicycle-related injuries seen in U.S. emergency departments.

Source: CDC (April 14, 2009).

Figure 10-1: Leading Causes of Death

Aged 1–24 years
Number of deaths = 39,086

- Unintentional injuries (38%)
- Homicide (13%)
- Suicide (12%)
- Cancer (7%)
- Heart disease (3%)
- All other causes (25%)

Aged 25–44 years
Number of deaths = 112,117

- Unintentional injuries (25%)
- Cancer (14%)
- Heart disease (12%)
- Suicide (11%)
- Homicide (6%)
- All other causes (32%)

Aged 45–64 years
Number of deaths = 493,376

- Cancer (32%)
- Heart disease (21%)
- Unintentional injuries (7%)
- Chronic lower respiratory diseases (4%)
- Chronic liver disease and cirrhosis (4%)
- All other causes (32%)

Aged 65 and over
Number of deaths = 1,796,620

- Heart disease (27%)
- Cancer (22%)
- Chronic lower respiratory diseases (7%)
- Stroke (6%)
- Alzheimer's disease (5%)
- All other causes (34%)

Source: National Vital Statistics System, Mortality (2011).

Exercise 10-17: *Multiple-choice question*

Which of the following activities would best target the cognitive domain to ensure that parents understand the new bicycle helmet program?

A. Watching a movie about bicycle maintenance—YES, this method would appeal to visual and auditory learners in a method that was entertaining.

B. A lecture and film about helmet use—NO, this only captures helmets, which is just one aspect of bike safety.

C. Role-playing activities—NO, this may not appeal to as many learners since it focuses on psychomotor or behavioral learning.

D. Hands-on practice with a variety of helmets—NO, this may not appeal to as many learners since it focuses on psychomotor or behavioral learning and only concentrates on the helmet aspect.

Exercise 10-18: *Multiple-choice question*

At the presentation, Janice provides information about the incidence of injury, the likelihood of injury, the severity of injury, as well as the simple steps that can be taken to protect health. Using this approach, she is applying which of the following?

A. Stages of Change Model—NO, she has not assessed the parents' stage of change or readiness to change behavior.

B. Transtheoretical Model—NO, she is not using a model that assesses readiness to change.

C. Health Belief Model—YES, this model best describes Janice's approach to promote a change in behavior.

D. Self-Efficacy Model—NO, she is not increasing individual confidence in a specific situation.

Exercise 10-19: *Multiple-choice question*

Providing this information to parents and teachers is

A. Primary prevention—YES

B. Secondary prevention—NO, she is not screening for disease.

C. Tertiary prevention—NO, she is not treating.

D. Health protection—NO

Exercise 10-20: *Multiple-choice question*

When Lisa uses the checklist to assess a child who has fallen off the monkey bars, she is engaging in:

A. Primary prevention—NO, this is preventative teaching.

B. Secondary prevention—YES, she is screening for injury.

C. Tertiary prevention—NO, she is not treating.

D. Health protection—NO

Exercise 10-21: *True or false*

A person who has had a concussion would show external evidence of a head injury such as a cut, bruise, or bump.

A. True

B. False

Exhibit 10-5: Answer Details

A person injured may not necessarily show evidence of a head injury. Signs and symptoms include:

- Appears dazed or stunned
- Is confused about events
- Answers questions slowly
- Repeats questions
- Can't recall events prior to the hit, bump, or fall
- Can't recall events after the hit, bump, or fall
- Loses consciousness (even briefly)
- Shows behavior or personality changes

Source: CDC (March 23, 2012).

Exercise 10-22: *Multiple-choice question*
A model that focuses on health promotion from an interpersonal level is:
A. The Health Belief Model—NO, this is from a personal point of view.
B. The Theory of Reasoned Action—YES
C. The Ecological Model—NO, this is from an environmental point of view.
D. Stages of Change—NO, this is a change model.

Exercise 10-23: *Multiple-choice question*
The perspective that an individual progresses through five levels related to readiness to change—precontemplation, contemplation, preparation, action, and maintenance—when adopting new health behaviors is part of which theory?
A. The Health Belief Model—NO, this is health promotion on an individual basis.
B. The Theory of Reasoned Action—NO, this is promotion of health on an interpersonal level.
C. The Ecological Model—NO, this is from an environmental point of view.
D. Stages of Change—YES

Exercise 10-24: *Multiple-choice question*
When Janice considers multiple levels of influence such as intrapersonal, interpersonal, institutional, community, and public policy when planning her health promotion program, she is using which of the following?
A. The Health Belief Model—NO, this is individual.
B. The Theory of Reasoned Action—NO, this is interpersonal.
C. The Ecological Model—YES
D. Stages of Change—NO, this describes the stages of change.

11

Disaster

Unfolding Case Study #1 Henry Baker

Henry Baker, RN, is a nurse who works for the American Red Cross and is responsible for coordinating the agency's health services responses to disasters in the region. On a day-to-day basis, he works with community partners to ensure emergency preparedness.

Exercise 11-1: *True or false*
The American Red Cross is a federal agency charged with the responsibility to coordinate responses to disasters.

A. True

B. False

Henry knows that disasters can be caused by natural events or by human-created events or factors, and in some cases can be caused simultaneously by both.

Exercise 11-2: *Fill-in*
Provide examples of each type of disaster:

Table 11-1

Natural Disasters	Human-Made Disasters	Both Natural and Human-Made

Exercise 11-3: *Fill-in*
A disaster is defined as:

_____

_____

_____

Answers to this chapter begin on page 266.

Exercise 11-4: *True or false*

Disasters create the most devastation in developed countries due to the population density and expansive infrastructure.

    A. True

    B. False

Henry works with community groups to provide disaster preparedness education. As part of this program, he goes to community centers, schools, and churches to provide disaster preparedness education. Generally, Henry begins his presentation by telling the attendees: "Every emergency has a health impact. It is important that everyone takes steps to minimize the impact of disaster on the health and well-being of our community." He continues by explaining the role of public health in emergency preparedness and management.

 eResource 11-1: To supplement this information, Henry shows the attendees a video, *Public Health's Role in Emergency Preparedness and Management*: http://youtu.be/R0z6FRH4dYY

Henry tells attendees that disaster management requires attention to the three phases of a disaster: Preparation, Response, and Recovery. "Today, we are focusing on *preparation* and the importance of creating a disaster plan. To be successful, the plan must be realistic, simple, and flexible."

Figure 11-1: Disaster Management Cycle

Recovery   Preparation

Response

As the presentation continues, Henry knows that a major barrier that he must overcome is to heighten awareness of the community's risk or vulnerability in the event of a disaster.

Answers to this chapter begin on page 266.

Exercise 11-5: *Multiple-choice question*

Henry believes that if he just "states the facts" about disaster, people will take steps to protect themselves. This is reflective of which health promotion theory or model?

    A. Health Belief Model

    B. Theory of Reason Action

    C. Social Learning

    D. Social Cognitive Theory

Exercise 11-6: *Multiple-choice question*

Conducting the disaster preparedness training is

    A. Primary prevention

    B. Secondary prevention

    C. Tertiary prevention

    D. Health protection

 eResource 11-2: Henry uses the following materials in his presentation:
- Disaster Preparedness From Ready.gov: http://youtu.be/7CTj5KZk7eg
- The Red Cross's Prepare Your Home and Family program: http://arcbrcr.org/#SITE and supplements his instruction with
- The Federal Emergency Management Agency's (FEMA) manual, *Are You Ready?*: http://goo.gl/FTWGJ

Henry tells the attendees that numerous agencies—federal, local, as well as non-governmental agencies (NGOs)—cooperate when disasters occur.

Exercise 11-7: *Select all that apply*

The following agencies participate in the event of a disaster in the United States:

- ❏ FEMA
- ❏ Red Cross
- ❏ Department of Health and Human Services
- ❏ National Institutes of Health
- ❏ United Nations
- ❏ Religious organizations
- ❏ Salvation Army
- ❏ Department of Defense (DoD)
- ❏ Food and Drug Administration (FDA)

 eResource 11-3: As part of his presentation, Henry provides each attendee a disaster preparedness checklist and family disaster preparation: http://goo.gl/HZv6t

During a community disaster preparedness program, a resident asks Henry, "I understand what you mean about the types of disasters that can occur, but what do you mean by *characteristics* of a disaster?"

Answers to this chapter begin on page 266.

Exercise 11-8: *Fill-in*

Describe the characteristics of a disaster that are considered when describing and preparing for a disaster.

1. _____

2. _____

3. _____

4. _____

5. _____

Henry uses this opportunity to return to the discussion about the Disaster Management Cycle. "There is another dimension to this cycle that can have significant impact on the risk of a disaster. Certainly, we cannot prevent hurricanes and tornadoes, but we can take proactive measures to try to *prevent* disasters—or at least minimize the impact."

Figure 11-2: Proactive Disaster Management

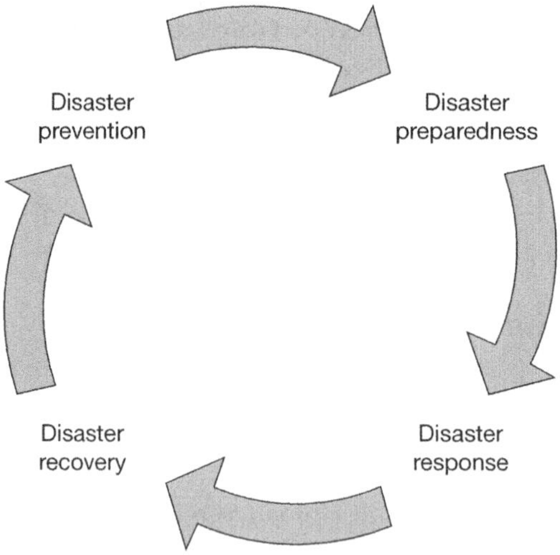

Henry asks the attendees to think about proactive measures that can be implemented to reduce or eliminate the risk of a disaster.

Exercise 11-9: *Fill-in*

What measures can be taken to prevent disasters?

_____

_____

_____

_____

Answers to this chapter begin on page 266.

Henry knows that it is important to be prepared and it should occur not only at the individual or family level and the community level, but also at the professional level.

Exercise 11-10: *Select all that apply*

To be professionally prepared for a disaster, Henry should have the following:

- ❑ Copy of nursing license
- ❑ Copy of his CPR and First-Aid Cards
- ❑ Disaster response training
- ❑ Family disaster plan
- ❑ Personal equipment (stethoscope, BP cuff, etc.)
- ❑ Cash
- ❑ Weather-appropriate clothing
- ❑ Record-keeping materials
- ❑ Mobile device with references/hard copy

Henry knows that the role of the nurse in disaster response is the identification and assessment of populations at risk because populations at risk have fewer resources and are less able to withstand and survive a disaster without physical harm. In addition, these populations tend to be physically isolated, disabled, or unable to access disaster services. Part of the strategic emergency planning process is to identify these individuals.

Exercise 11-11: *Select all that apply*

Which of the following populations should be identified as particularly *at risk* for disaster planning purposes?

- ❑ The elderly living in the community
- ❑ Children living in the community
- ❑ The mentally ill
- ❑ The elderly living in senior housing
- ❑ Previous disaster or trauma victims
- ❑ Immigrants
- ❑ Minority groups
- ❑ The homeless
- ❑ Persons with disabilities
- ❑ Non–English-speaking or refugees
- ❑ Persons living alone

Answers to this chapter begin on page 266.

Exercise 11-12: *Select all that apply*
Disaster victims include:

❏ Direct casualties

❏ Indirect casualties

❏ Displaced persons

❏ Refugees

The nurse's role in a disaster response frequently involves triaging victims and prioritizing care. To prepare for this role, Henry attended special training.

 eResource 11-3: As part of the training, he watches the START Triage Basics video: http://youtu.be/9QHDs10e-G0

Henry is responsible for coordinating training for community volunteers to be available to respond in the event of an incident involving mass casualties.

 eResource 11-4: To conduct this training, Henry uses training materials from FEMA's Community Emergency Response Team program:
■ CERT—START—RPM (Part 1): http://youtu.be/73kJ-4gEsnA
■ CERT—START—RPM (Part 2): http://youtu.be/4NHSAZW0d5Y
■ CERT Triage: Handling Mass Casualty Situations training video: http://youtu.be/LUusRUsfKAA

Henry and his nurse colleagues use the JumpSTART triage tool when working as the triage nurses in a disaster situation. Using this tool serves as an effective guide to quickly screen victims, prioritize care, provide the care they need, and clear the area.

 eResource 11-5: JumpSTART
■ Adult: http://goo.gl/kEvmF
■ Pediatric: http://goo.gl/u8gu7

Exercise 11-13: *Multiple-choice question*
The first thing to do when arriving at a mass casualty site is
A. Assess casualties
B. See who else is around to help
C. Check safety of the environment
D. Call for help

Exercise 11-14: *Matching*
Match the color with the appropriate triage status.
A. Red   _____ Urgent; second priority
B. Yellow   _____ Dying or dead
C. Green   _____ Most urgent; first priority
D. Black   _____ Third priority

Henry knows that he and his team will be serving a diverse population that includes newly immigrated minorities, and it is important to provide culturally competent care even in emergency situations. The team is interested in becoming more culturally competent and better able to work effectively in high-stress, cross-cultural situations.

 eResource 11-6: To build this competency, Henry and his team of volunteers receive the following training:
- Cultural Competency Curriculum for Disaster Preparedness: http://goo.gl/cwb0a
- RESPOND TOOL for emergency responders: Culturally Competent History Taking in a Crisis http://goo.gl/9GnZB

As part of his plan for the recovery phase of the disaster, Henry wants to make sure that he has contact information for available resources and services for the victims. He realizes that in addition to providing linkage to the U.S. Department of Housing and Urban Development and the International Relief Services; he also must provide linkage for mental health services. Henry knows that posttraumatic stress disorders (PTSD) and delayed stress reactions (DSR) are common during the aftermath of disasters. PTSD and DSR affect both the victims and caregivers. He also knows that the longer it takes to repair and clean up, the more psychological effects emerge and the longer the recovery takes.

Exercise 11-15: *Fill-in*
What are the symptoms of PTSD?

_____

_____

_____

Exercise 11-16: *Fill-in*
When encountering a person suffering from PTSD, what should the nurse consider first?

_____

_____

_____

Unfolding Case Study #2 Volunteer Emergency Responder

Daniel and Sarah are RNs working as volunteers with the Community Emergency Response Triage (CERT) in a rural community in southwestern Jefferson County in Kentucky. They receive a call that there has been a train derailment involving a chemical spill and numerous casualties. The disaster is reported to be a Level 3 HazMat Alert with forced evacuations within a 1-mile radius.

Answers to this chapter begin on page 266.

As they prepare a triage station to process victims for transport to the local emergency department, they are told that the chemical is butadiene. The news report released had the following information, "the Paducah & Louisville Railway train consisted of 39 cars, and eight of them derailed . . . the car carrying butadiene was upside down. The derailed tanker car has a capacity of 30,000 gallons. Officials did not immediately know how much butadiene it was carrying" (Gazaway, 2012). Daniel quickly refers to the Wireless Information System for Emergency Responders (WISER) and looks up butadiene.

 eResource 11-7: Both Daniel and Sarah have WISER downloaded on their mobile device: http://wiser.nlm.nih.gov

One of the first things that Daniel and Sarah learned in their training as CERT team responders is to ensure a safe working environment for themselves. What are the considerations for personal protective equipment for them?

Exercise 11-17: *True or false*
There is no significant risk for secondary contamination for rescuers and first responders caring for individuals exposed to butadiene.

    A. True

    B. False

Exercise 11-18: *Fill-in*
What is the key information provided in WISER related to butadiene?

_____

_____

Exercise 11-19: *Multiple-choice question*
What are the cardiovascular effects of acute exposure to butadiene?

    A. Tachycardia

    B. Bradycardia

    C. Atrial arrhythmias

    D. Angina

Exercise 11-20: *Fill-in*
What is the treatment for respiratory exposure to butadiene?

_____

_____

One of the victims brought to the triage station is reported to have ingested a substantial amount of butadiene. Sarah quickly looks up the treatment protocol on her device.

Answers to this chapter begin on page 266.

Exercise 11-21: *Fill-in*

What is the treatment for oral ingestion of butadiene?

_____

_____

Sarah prepares the victim for gastric lavage. She knows that this procedure must be done on site because it is important to remove the ingested substance to decrease systemic absorption.

Exercise 11-22: *Multiple-choice question*

The proper patient position for the gastric lavage procedure is:

    A. Right lateral with head level

    B. Left lateral with head level

    C. Right lateral with head at about 15 degrees

    D. Left lateral with head about 15 degrees

After completing the gastric lavage, Sarah and Daniel prepare the patient for transport to the hospital.

Unfolding Case Study #3   Bioterrorism

Louise McNeil is a retired nurse who volunteers for the local American Red Cross. She participates regularly in disaster preparedness trainings and drills. She realizes that there is considerable concern regarding bioterrorism and stays up to date on proper procedures and protocols associated with this emerging threat to public safety. Louise knows that a nurse's role includes being alert to signs of possible terrorist activity and being prepared to follow the disaster plan and provide direct care.

Exercise 11-23: *True or false*

Biological warfare has only recently emerged as a military weapon.

    A. True

    B. False

Louise knows that there are three categories of biological agents utilized in biological warfare, and Category A poses the most threat to national security and the public's health.

Exercise 11-24: *Fill-in*

Why do Category A biological agents pose the most serious threat to national security and the public's health?

_____

_____

_____

Answers to this chapter begin on page 266.

Exercise 11-25: *Select all that apply*

Which of the following are considered Category A biological agents?

❑ Typhus fever (*Rickettsia prowazekii*)

❑ Anthrax (*Bacillus anthracis*)

❑ Botulism (*Clostridium botulinum* toxin)

❑ Ricin toxin (from castor beans)

❑ Plague (*Yersinia pestis*)

❑ Smallpox (*variola major*)

❑ Glanders (*Burkholderia mallei*)

❑ Melioidosis (*Burkholderia pseudomallei*)

❑ Psittacosis (*Chlamydia psittaci*)

❑ Tularemia (*Francisella tularensis*)

❑ Viral hemorrhagic fevers (filoviruses and arenaviruses)

The role of the nurse in preparation for a biological attack includes participation in planning and preparation for immediate response to a bioterrorist event. She must be able to identify potential biological agents for bioterrorism and report promptly any observed or suspected bioterrorism activity to the local health department. These activities are proactive in nature with the goal of *preventing* a bioterrorist event (see Figure 11-2).

Exercise 11-26: *Fill-in*

Describe primary prevention measures that Louise could participate in.

_____

_____

_____

As part of the *response phase*, Louise knows she must promptly participate in measures to contain and control the spread of infections resulting from bioterrorist activity.

Exercise 11-27: *Fill-in*

Describe the secondary prevention activities that Louise could put into place during the response phase.

_____

_____

_____

_____

Answers to this chapter begin on page 266.

Exercise 11-28: *True or false*

For individuals who have been exposed to anthrax, prophylactic antibiotic therapy is of no therapeutic value.

    A. True

    B. False

Exercise 11-29: *True or false*

Anthrax exposure can mimic symptoms of a cold or flu.

    A. True

    B. False

Exercise 11-30: *Fill-in*

Describe tertiary prevention activities that Louise could put into place during the recovery phase.

_____

_____

_____

_____

Answers

Exercise 11-1: *True or false*

The American Red Cross is a federal agency charged with the responsibility to coordinate responses to disasters.

 A. True

 B. False, partners with other agencies to assist in disasters.

Exhibit 11-1: Answer Details

"The American Red Cross exists to provide compassionate care to those in need. Our network of generous donors, volunteers, and employees share a mission of preventing and relieving suffering, here at home and around the world, through five key service areas: (a) Disaster relief, (b) Supporting America's military families, (c) Health and safety training and education, (d) Lifesaving blood and (e) International humanitarian services."

Source: Red Cross (2012).

Exercise 11-2: *Fill-in*

Provide examples of each type of disaster:

Table 11-2

Natural Disasters	Human-Made Disasters	Both Natural and Human-Made
Hurricanes Tornados Earthquakes Volcanic eruptions Landslides Monsoons Tsunami	Industrial accidents Construction accidents Transportation accidents Nuclear accidents Oil rig/mining accidents Terrorism	Floods following storms (caused by deforestation; levees failing; overbuilding on natural flood plains, etc., e.g., Katrina)

Exercise 11-3: *Fill-in*

A disaster is defined as:

"An event in which a community undergoes severe danger and incurs, or is threatened to incur, such losses to persons and/or property that the resources available within the community are exceeded. In disasters, resources from beyond the local jurisdiction, that is state or federal level, are required to meet the disaster demands" (Drabek, 1996, pp. 2–4).

Exercise 11-4: *True or false*

Disasters create the most devastation in developed countries due to the population density and expansive infrastructure.

A. True

B. False

Exhibit 11-2: Answer Details

Disasters create the most devastation in developing countries because there are fewer resources available, there is less ability for warning and preparation, homes or buildings are less sturdy, and governmental and social support systems lack resources to respond.

Exercise 11-5: *Multiple-choice question*

Henry believes that if he just "states the facts" about disaster, people will take steps to protect themselves. This is reflective of which health promotion theory or model?

A. Health Belief Model—NO, this is about individuals self-focusing on their health.

B. Theory of Reason Action—YES, self-protection would be the most likely reasonable thing to do.

C. Social learning—NO, this is a learning theory, not a health belief theory or model.

D. Social cognitive theory—NO, this is a learning theory, not a health belief theory or model.

Exercise 11-6: *Multiple-choice question*

Conducting the disaster preparedness training is:

A. Primary prevention—YES, primary prevention is proactive, frequently in the form of education.

B. Secondary prevention—NO, this is looking for ways to decrease the potential risk.

C. Tertiary prevention—NO, this is an intervention focused upon restoration or rehabilitation.

D. Health protection—NO, this is focused upon the individual.

Exercise 11-7: *Select all that apply*

The following agencies participate in the event of a disaster in the United States:

☒ **FEMA**

☒ **Red Cross**

☐ Department of Health and Human Services

❑ National Institutes of Health

❑ United Nations

☒ **Religious organizations**

☒ **Salvation Army**

❑ Department of Defense (DoD)

❑ FDA

Exercise 11-8: *Fill-in*

Describe the characteristics of a disaster that are considered when describing and preparing for a disaster.

 1. Length of forewarning

 2. Magnitude of impact

 3. Geographical scope of impact

 4. Duration of impact

 5. Speed of onset

Exercise 11-9: *Fill-in*

What measures can be taken to prevent disasters?

Preventative measure can include enforcement of safety and security measures (e.g., aviation regulations, oil rigs regulations, homeland security, etc.); regular maintenance of key infrastructure (e.g., repair of levees, dams); educated and empowered citizenry.

Exercise 11-10: *Select all that apply*

To be professionally prepared for a disaster, Henry should have the following:

☒ **Copy of nursing license**

☒ **Copy of CPR and First-Aid Cards**

☒ **Disaster response training**

❑ Family disaster plan

☒ **Personal equipment (stethoscope, BP cuff, etc.)**

☒ **Cash**

☒ **Weather-appropriate clothing**

☒ **Record-keeping materials**

☒ **Mobile device with references/hard copy**

Exercise 11-11: *Select all that apply*

Which of the following populations should be identified as particularly *at risk* for disaster planning purposes?

☒ **The elderly living in the community**

❑ Children living in the community

☒ **The mentally ill**

☐ The elderly living in senior housing

☒ **Previous disaster or trauma victims**

☐ Immigrants

☐ Minority groups

☒ **The homeless**

☒ **Persons with disabilities**

☒ **Non–English-speaking or refugees**

☒ **Persons living alone**

Exercise 11-12: *Select all that apply*

Disaster victims include:

☒ **Direct casualties**

☒ **Indirect casualties**

☒ **Displaced persons**

☒ **Refugees**

Exercise 11-13: *Multiple-choice question*

The first thing to do when arriving at a mass casualty site is

A. Assess casualties—NO, this is not the safest intervention

B. See who else is around to help—NO

C. **Check safety of the environment—YES, you need to make sure it works.**

D. Call for help—NO, this has already been done.

Exercise 11-14: *Matching*

Match the color with the appropriate triage status.

A. Red	**B**	Urgent; second priority
B. Yellow	**D**	Dying or dead
C. Green	**A**	Most urgent; first priority
D. Black	**C**	Third priority

Exercise 11-15: *Fill-in*

What are the symptoms for PTSD?

- **Symptoms of intrusive memories (flashbacks, dreams, etc.)**
- **Symptoms of avoidance and emotional numbing (trying to avoid thinking or talking about the traumatic event, avoiding activities that one once enjoyed, memory problems, difficulty concentrating, hopelessness, problems with relationships)**
- **Symptoms of anxiety and increased emotional arousal (irritability or anger, guilt or shame, self-destructive behavior such as drinking too much, sleep disturbances, easily startled or frightened, hearing or seeing things that aren't there) (Mayo Clinic, 2011)**

Exercise 11-16: *Fill-in*

When encountering a person suffering from PTSD, what should the nurse consider first?

The nurse should assess for safety and level of risk for harm to oneself or others. The priority is to link the person to mental health support services immediately; ideally to bring the mental health service to the person or to "walk the person" to the service, if this is possible.

Exercise 11-17: *True or false*

There is no significant risk for secondary contamination for rescuers and first responders caring for individuals exposed to butadiene.

A. True

B. False

Exhibit 11-3: Answer Details

While persons exposed to butadiene gas pose no risk of secondary contamination to rescuers, those whose skin or clothing is heavily contaminated with liquid butadiene can secondarily contaminate response personnel by direct contact or through rapidly evaporating gas. It is advisable for Daniel and Sarah to wear personal protective equipment (gowns and gloves). (National Library of Medicine, 2012).

Exercise 11-18: *Fill-in*

What is the key information provided in WISER related to butadiene?

Butadiene Key Info:

- **GASES—FLAMMABLE (Unstable)**
- **EXTREMELY FLAMMABLE**

Exhibit 11-4: Answer Details

[Pathway: WISER (http://goo.gl/9nE3s) → select "substance list" → enter "Butadiene" into the search field → select "Key Info"]

Exercise 11-19: *Multiple-choice question*

What are the cardiovascular effects of acute exposure to butadiene?

A. Tachycardia—NO, it does not speed up the rate of the heart.

B. Bradycardia—YES

C. Atrial arrhythmias—NO, it does not produce a dysrhythmic beat.

D. Angina—NO, it does not produce pain.

Exhibit 11-5: Answer Details

[Pathway: WISER (http://goo.gl/9nE3s) → select "substance list" → enter "Butadiene" into the search field → select "Medical" → select "Health Effects"]

Exercise 11-20: *Fill-in*

What is the treatment for respiratory exposure to butadiene?

INHALATION EXPOSURE: Move patient to fresh air. Monitor for respiratory distress. If cough or difficulty breathing develops, evaluate for respiratory tract irritation, bronchitis, or pneumonitis. Administer oxygen and assist ventilation as required. Treat bronchospasm with inhaled beta-2 agonist and oral or parenteral corticosteroids (WISER http://goo.gl/yn6uY).

Exercise 11-21: *Fill-in*

What is the treatment for oral ingestion of butadiene?

A. **"GASTRIC LAVAGE: Consider after ingestion of a potentially life-threatening amount of poison if it can be performed soon after ingestion (generally within 1 hour). Protect airway by placement in Trendelenburg and left lateral decubitus position or by endotracheal intubation. Control any seizures first. (a) CONTRAINDICATIONS: Loss of airway protective reflexes or decreased level of consciousness in unintubated patients; following ingestion of corrosives; hydrocarbons (high aspiration potential); patients at risk of hemorrhage or gastrointestinal perforation; and trivial or nontoxic ingestion.**

B. **ACTIVATED CHARCOAL: Administer charcoal as a slurry (240 mL water/30 g charcoal). Usual dose: 25 to 100 g in adults/adolescents, 25 to 50 g in children (1–12 years), and 1 g/kg in infants less than 1 year old.**

C. **Butadiene is only a mild irritant and its primary toxicity is CNS depression and anesthesia in high concentrations (shown in animal studies). Treatment of serious cases would involve support of respiratory function. (a) No serious human exposures have yet been reported" (WISER http://goo.gl/yn6uY).**

Exercise 11-22: *Multiple-choice question*

The proper patient position for the gastric lavage procedure is:

A. Right lateral with head level—NO, this is fighting against too much gravity.

B. Left lateral with head level—NO, this may cause them to aspirate.

C. Right lateral with head at about 15 degrees—NO, the right side decreases the chance of proper placement of the tube in the stomach.

D. **Left lateral with head about 15 degrees—YES**

Exhibit 11-6: Answer Details

This position decreases passage of gastric contents into the duodenum during the gastric lavage procedure.

Exercise 11-23: *True or false*
Biological warfare has only recently emerged as a military weapon.
A. True
B. False

Exhibit 11-7: Answer Details

> Biological warfare has been used for more than 2,000 years; it was used during sieges in the Middle Ages, smallpox blankets were given to Native Americans, and mustard gas was utilized by Germany in World War I and by Japan in World War II.

Exercise 11-24: *Fill-in*
Why do Category A biological agents pose the most serious threat to national security and the public's health?
Category A biological agents pose the greatest threat because they can be easily disseminated or transmitted from person to person, result in high mortality rates, and have the potential for major public health impact and might cause public panic and social disruption.

Exercise 11-25: *Select all that apply*
Which of the following are considered Category A biological agents?
❑ Typhus fever (*Rickettsia prowazekii*)
☒ **Anthrax (*Bacillus anthracis*)**
☒ **Botulism (*Clostridium botulinum* toxin)**
❑ Ricin toxin (from castor beans)
☒ **Plague (*Yersinia pestis*)**
☒ **Smallpox (variola major)**
❑ Glanders (*Burkholderia mallei*)
❑ Melioidosis (*Burkholderia pseudomallei*)
❑ Psittacosis (*Chlamydia psittaci*)
☒ **Tularemia (*Francisella tularensis*)**
☒ **Viral hemorrhagic fevers (filoviruses and arenaviruses)**

Exercise 11-26: *Fill-in*
Describe primary prevention measures that Louise could participate in.
Primary prevention measures:
- **Bioterrorism drills**
- **Preparation of vaccines and antibiotics for prophylaxis**
- **Bioterrorism planning**
- **Design response plan**

- **Assess and locate facilities that have level I, II, III, and IV biosafety gear**
- **Identify chain of command**
- **Define nursing roles**
- **Set up protocols**
- **Educate the public**

Exercise 11-27: *Fill-in*
Describe secondary prevention activities that Louise could put into place during the response phase.
Secondary prevention measures:
- **Early recognition**
- **Activation of bioterrorism response plan**
- **Immediate implementation of infection control and containment measures**
- **Decontamination**
- **Environmental disinfection**
- **Protective equipment**
- **Community education or notification**
- **Quarantines**

Exercise 11-28: *True or false*
For individuals who have been exposed to anthrax, prophylactic antibiotic therapy is of no therapeutic value.
A. True
B. False

Exhibit 11-8: Answer Details

Antibiotics are recommended for all three types of anthrax. Early identification and treatment are important. Prevention after exposure but not yet sick: Antibiotics (such as ciprofloxacin, levofloxacin, doxycycline, or penicillin) combined with the anthrax vaccine to prevent anthrax infection. Treatment after infection: Usually a 60-day course of antibiotics. Success depends on the type of anthrax and how soon treatment begins.

Exercise 11-29: *True or false*
Anthrax exposure can mimic symptoms of a cold or flu.
A. True
B. False

Exhibit 11-9: Answer Details

Symptoms (generally present within 7 days) depend on type:

- Cutaneous: small sore develops into a blister. Blister develops into an ulcer with black area in the center. All are painless.

- Gastrointestinal: Nausea, loss of appetite, bloody diarrhea, and fever, followed by bad stomach pain.

- Inhalation: Cold or flulike symptoms. Can include a sore throat, mild fever, and muscle aches. Later symptoms include cough, chest discomfort and shortness of breath, tiredness, and muscle aches. (PLEASE NOTE: Do not assume that just because a person has cold or flu symptoms they have inhalation anthrax.)

Exercise 11-30: *Fill-in*

Describe tertiary prevention activities that Louise could put into place during the recovery phase.

Tertiary prevention measures:

- **Rehabilitation of survivors**
- **Monitoring medication regimens and referrals**
- **Evaluation of the effectiveness and timeliness of the bioterrorism plan**
- **Recovery assistance**

Violence and Abuse

Unfolding Case Study #1 ▧ Child Abuse

Johanna Milton, RN, is a parish nurse working in a rural community near Bakersfield, California. She started working as a parish nurse about 25 years ago when the implementation of diagnosis-related groups led to patients being discharged from the hospital more quickly and much sicker. The families were overwhelmed with these new caregiving responsibilities, so the parish decided to hire Johanna and three other nurses to provide faith-based, supportive nursing services. Johanna loves her job and has over the years established deep connections within this close-knit community. The people of the parish trust her and have come to rely on her guidance and support.

Exercise 12-1: *Select all that apply*
The functions of the parish nurse include:

- ❑ Financial advisor
- ❑ Guardian
- ❑ Personal health counseling
- ❑ Health education
- ❑ Direct patient care
- ❑ Liaison with social service agencies
- ❑ Legal advisor
- ❑ Facilitator
- ❑ Pastoral care
- ❑ Advocate

While Johanna was finishing a home visit to an elderly parish member who lives in a trailer park, a neighbor, Alice Jones, pulled her aside and asked for her advice. She tells Johanna that she has been caring for two young boys, Steve and Mark Williams, for a week and she doesn't know what to do. As the story unfolds, Johanna learns that the two boys had been at Alice's home playing with her children. At the end of the day, the boys left to go home. Shortly afterwards, the boys returned and told Alice that their house was gone. Sure enough, the trailer was gone. Alice has let the boys stay with her hoping that their parents, Martin and Madeline, would return. "It's been a week, Johanna! And not a word from them. . . . I just don't know what I should do."

Exercise 12-2: *Multiple-choice question*

The best response for Johanna to give is

        A. "It's only been a week; why not keep the boys a little longer until the parents come back."

        B. "You should go to the police and file a missing persons report for Martin and Madeline."

        C. "This is neglect, a form of child abuse, and by law must be reported to the authorities."

        D. "Do you have the phone numbers of any of the Williams' friends and relatives? Let's try calling them."

Exercise 12-3: *True or false*

Since Alice is a responsible adult and is caring for Mark and Steve, Johanna has an ethical but not legal responsibility to report the situation.

        A. True

        B. False

 eResource 12-1: For current information regarding Mandatory Reporters of Child Abuse and Neglect: Summary of State Laws, Johanna visits: http://goo.gl/avVnR

Johanna goes with Alice into her trailer and uses her cell phone to call child protective services (CPS). She waits with Alice for the CPS worker to arrive. While she is there, she observes the two brothers playing with Alice's son. Mark and Steve appear happy and very attached to one another. The boys are very affectionate toward Alice, stopping their play when they had entered the trailer to give Alice a spontaneous hug. The boys are both thin and small for their reported ages of 5 and 6. Their clothes are old and worn but clean (thanks to Alice). Although it is the middle of October, the boys are barefoot. When asked why, the eldest responds, "Because they're too tight." A cursory exam does not reveal any outward evidence of physical abuse.

Exercise 12-4: *Fill-in*

If Johanna suspects child abuse, what else should she be assessing? What other signs and symptoms would indicate abuse?

_____

_____

_____

Answers to this chapter begin on page 285.

As Johanna watches the boys play, she remembers a child abuse awareness seminar she attended last year. At that time, the presenter spoke about behavior changes to watch for in children that can provide clues about abuse (Child Welfare Information Gateway, 2007).

Exercise 12-5: *Fill-in*
List the behavior changes to watch for in children that can provide clues about abuse.

Table 12-1

Behavior Changes Associated With Abuse	
Physical abuse	
Neglect	
Sexual abuse	
Emotional abuse	

Johanna reflects on the events of the day and thinks how things for the two boys could have been different if more community support and programs were available.

Exercise 12-6: *Select all that apply*
Which of the following would be utilized as primary prevention strategies for child abuse or neglect?

❑ Teenage pregnancy prevention programs
❑ Parenting classes
❑ Reporting requirements
❑ Family strengthening programs
❑ Community awareness
❑ Incarceration

 eResource 12-2: Child Welfare Information Gateway: http://goo.gl/ENroP

Johanna realizes that child abuse and neglect is a societal issue that is very complex. She believes that any approach to address the problems must be multilevel and focus on individual, relationship, community, and societal factors.

Unfolding Case Study #2 ▰ Elder Abuse

Ferne Henway is a home health care nurse, who is assigned to visit Mr. Victor Morelli, newly discharged from the hospital, where he was treated for exacerbation of his congestive heart failure. Victor has trouble getting around and needs to use a walker to ambulate. His recent hospitalization made him realize that he can no longer live alone. He needs help with his day-to-day activities. In addition, he can no longer go up and down the stairs in his two-story home. Fortunately his home has a full bath and bedroom on the first floor, so he has moved his bedroom to the first floor.

Victor's 20-year-old granddaughter, Nadia, has agreed to move in with him. Victor is very relieved that Nadia has agreed to stay with him. He could not bear the thought of leaving his beloved home of 45 years.

Nadia welcomed the opportunity to move in and help her grandfather because she had to move out of her previous apartment because the landlord sold the building, which is now slated to be converted to condominiums. It seems like a perfect solution for both. Ferne arrives for the initial home visit.

Exercise 12-7: *Fill-in*
What would be the most important element to assess in the home environment?

_____

_____

_____

Ferne knows that when a nurse enters the home, he or she is a guest and that the home care services offered can be accepted or rejected by the client. The first home visit can set the stage for success or failure, and initial assessment of the client, the support system, and the home environment is critical. Ferne knows that it is important to establish a mutually agreed upon plan of care. One way to formalize this process is to establish a client contract. An important first step in this endeavor is to engage Mr. Morelli in a discussion regarding his priorities.

Exercise 12-8: *Fill-in*
What strategies would the nurse consider to develop a trusting relationship during the first home visit?

_____

_____

_____

Exercise 12-9: *Fill-in*
What should be included in a client contract?

_____

_____

_____

_____

_____

Victor's granddaughter, Nadia, is present for the first home visit and seems genuinely concerned and interested in providing good care for her grandfather. She

Answers to this chapter begin on page 285.

asks appropriate questions about Victor's medications and dietary restrictions. She asks Ferne, "Should he take his Lanoxin before or after he has breakfast?"

Exercise 12-10: *Multiple-choice question*
The best response to Nadia's question is:
- A. "It doesn't matter when he takes his medication, just as long as he takes it the same time each day."
- B. "It is best that he takes his medication after he has eaten something."
- C. "You should check his heart rate every morning before taking this medication."
- D. B and C
- E. All of the above

At subsequent home visits, everything seems to be going well by Victor's report. His vital signs and weight remain stable. Nadia is not present for several home visits. Ferne notices that Nadia hasn't been present for the last four home visits. She casually remarks, "So how is everything going? How is Nadia? I haven't seen her for a while." Victor tells Ferne that Nadia is working two jobs and is very busy. "But, she fixes my meals and takes good care of me," he reports.

One day, Ferne notices that Victor has a bruise on the right side of his head. She asks him about it, and he tells her that he tripped and fell. Ferne examines Victor. She notes that he also has bruising on his right upper arm, hip, and knee. She assesses his balance.

 eResource 12-3: Ferne consults her resources:
- Balance Assessment Handbook: http://goo.gl/CWZqk
- Fall Risk Assessment: http://goo.gl/x5oie
- Morse Fall Scale: http://goo.gl/2ilXC

Ferne continues with her assessment of Victor.

Exercise 12-11: *Fill-in*
When assessing a patient following a head injury, what should Ferne consider?

_____

_____

_____

Exercise 12-12: *Fill-in*
What environmental factors or modifications should be considered to reduce the risk of falling?

_____

_____

_____

_____

Answers to this chapter begin on page 285.

Ferne notes that all of the recommended measures to reduce risk of falling are in place. She thinks about the bruising on Victor's upper arm. She remembers a recent conference she attended where she saw a presentation by Ronald Chez, MD, FACOG, entitled "Elder Abuse: An Overview for the Clinician."

 eResource 12-4: Elder Abuse: http://goo.gl/yTSCx

Ferne knows that elders, like Victor, are at risk for abuse and that often they do not report it because they are dependent upon their caregiver or perhaps in fear of the caregiver. Ferne remembers that Victor was desperate to stay in his home and very grateful that Nadia was willing to come live with him. Ferne decides that she would like to screen Victor for abuse.

 eResource 12-5: To guide her next steps, Ferne consults the following:
- Risk Assessment Tools for Elder Abuse: http://goo.gl/YQ6IF
- National Guideline Clearinghouse Standard of Practice: http://goo.gl/gXcZd

Exercise 12-13: *Select all that apply*
Which of the following statements about elder abuse are correct?

☐ Elder abuse can be physical, verbal, financial, or psychological/emotional.

☐ Elder abuse is a major public health problem, occurring in approximately 30% to 40% of the elderly population.

☐ The majority of elder abuse is committed by nonfamilial caregivers.

☐ Elder abuse is underreported.

Exercise 12-14: *Fill-in*
What should be included in a nursing assessment for elder abuse?

_____

_____

_____

_____

After speaking with Victor some more about the fall, Ferne can see that Victor is adamant that he does not want to leave his home. He is reluctant to talk more about his recent fall. Nevertheless, Ferne wants to follow up with Nadia. Ferne knows that it is important to approach Nadia directly to address her concerns about Victor's safety. She also realizes that caregiving is hard and wants to provide support to Nadia.

Answers to this chapter begin on page 285.

Exercise 12-15: *Fill-in*

What strategies would the nurse consider to develop a trusting and supportive relationship with Nadia?

_____

_____

_____

Ferne makes it a point to make a home visit when Nadia is home and sits with her privately in the kitchen. "I am glad to have this opportunity to chat with you. How are you?" The two engage in a conversation that eventually leads to the topic of caregiving and caregiving burden. Nadia admits that she is stressed with working two jobs and caring for Victor. "Sometimes I get impatient with him . . . he moves so slow and it takes forever to get anything done." She admits that one time, she grabbed his arm and shoved him to get him to move faster . . . one time, he fell. "I didn't mean for it to happen."

Exercise 12-16: *Multiple-choice question*

How should Ferne respond?

     A. "What you did is elder abuse and is against the law."

     B. Ferne should not confront Nadia. She should leave and report the incident to the authorities.

     C. "Caregiving is hard. There is help available that can lighten the load for you."

     D. "You should reach out to your church to get some help in caring for Victor."

Ferne knows that it is important that she work toward establishing trust with Nadia and to use a nonjudgmental approach in addressing this matter. She also needs to develop a plan of care to help support both Victor and Nadia.

Exercise 12-17: *Fill-in*

What are the nursing care priorities and interventions?

_____

_____

_____

_____

Answers to this chapter begin on page 285.

Unfolding Case Study #3 Intimate Partner Violence

Monica and Rachel are senior nursing students participating in a community health fair. Gwen is the public health nurse organizing the health fair. Since it is October, the focus is on women's health issues, particularly breast cancer awareness and domestic violence awareness. Since it is Domestic Violence Awareness Month, Gwen asks the students to review the following information so that they can be prepared. "I always use health fairs as a good opportunity to do a little case finding. I take every opportunity to educate about domestic violence."

eResource 12-6: Domestic Abuse Screening:
- HITS Screening Tool: http://goo.gl/61jWa
- American Congress of Obstetricians and Gynecologists screening questions: http://goo.gl/XHsM2
- CDC Publication: Intimate Partner Violence and Sexual Violence Victimization Assessment http://goo.gl/r24Wd

Gwen has also asked Monica and Rachel to do blood pressure screenings. "Doing blood pressure screenings gets people in the door. Everybody wants to get their blood pressure checked. Once you have them in the chair . . . you have a captive audience. So use that to assess and teach!" Monica and Rachel are looking forward to the experience.

Exercise 12-18: *Multiple-choice question*
Doing blood pressure screenings at the health fair is:
- A. Primary prevention
- B. Secondary prevention
- C. Tertiary prevention
- D. Health promotion

As they prepare for the event, Monica and Rachel review their health education materials to ensure that these are appropriate for the audience they expect.

Exercise 12-19: *Fill-in*
What factors should be considered when selecting patient education material?

_____

_____

_____

Monica wants to make sure that they bring referral information along as well. She remembers that the instructor told the class that referral is an essential requirement of all screening programs. "Remember class, the purpose of screening is to identify individuals with disease *before* they have signs and symptoms of the disease to allow *early* intervention and treatment. So. . . referral is absolutely essential. It is unethical not to provide this referral," the instructor had told the class.

Answers to this chapter begin on page 285.

eResource 12-7: To help the students understand screening tests, the instructor had shown the class the National Library of Medicine's publication *What You Should Know About Screening Tests*: http://goo.gl/DuMRy

Exercise 12-20: *Select all that apply*
The World Health Organization has published guidelines regarding screening tests and strongly urges that screenings are conducted only when there is demonstrated value in doing so. These criteria include which of the following?

❑ Screenings should be done only for diseases with serious consequences so that there is a clear health benefit.

❑ There must be a sufficiently reliable and safe test method.

❑ Screenings must occur on a regular basis in order to prevent disease (screenings do not *prevent* disease, screenings permit *early detection* and *early treatment*).

❑ There must be an effective treatment proven to be more successful when started before symptoms occur.

❑ There should be neutral information available so that individuals can decide for themselves whether or not to have a screening test.

As the health fair progresses, a woman approaches the two students and asks for her blood pressure to be checked. Monica willingly obliges. As she takes the woman's blood pressure, she engages in a casual conversation and learns that the woman's name is Veronica. Veronica's blood pressure is 118/78—well within the normal range. While taking Veronica's blood pressure, Monica notices bruising on her arm, which appears to be from someone grabbing her arm. She asks Veronica about it. Veronica laughs nervously, but offers no information.

Exercise 12-21: *Fill-in*
What should Monica do next?

_____

_____

_____

Monica should ask Veronica the following questions:
"I notice you have a number of bruises; did someone do this to you? Are you afraid at home? Do you have a safety plan?" She should offer her information regarding domestic abuse, particularly hotline information.

Exercise 12-22: *Select all that apply*
Monica knows that frequently a woman will remain in an abusive relationship because she believes that:

❑ her partner will change

❑ she is partly to blame for the abuse

Answers to this chapter begin on page 285.

❑ if she leaves, he will escalate the abuse

❑ she has no place to go

❑ she can help her abuser

Monica knows that it is important that she be supportive and nonjudgmental in her communication with Veronica (Centers for Disease Control and Prevention, 2009).

Exercise 12-23: *Fill-in*

What can Monica say to communicate caring and support for Veronica?

_____

_____

_____

■ Pay attention to nonverbal communication; body language. Be nonjudgmental.

■ Treat Veronica with respect; convey to her that she deserves to be treated with respect.

■ Listen actively.

■ Reassure Veronica that she is not to blame for being battered or mistreated and she is not the cause of his behavior.

■ Convey concern about her safety.

Monica spends some time talking with Veronica and shares information about available resources for victims of domestic abuse. She talks to Veronica about developing a safety plan.

Exercise 12-24: *Fill-in*

What should be included in a safety plan?

_____

_____

_____

_____

Monica provides Veronica with additional information regarding a safety plan.

ⓔ **eResource 12-8:** Safety Planning Tool: http://goo.gl/OViND

Before Veronica leaves, Monica tells her, "Please remember, there are resources and supports available for you." She provides hotline information to Veronica.

ⓔ **eResource 12-9:** Toll-Free Domestic Violence Hotlines: http://goo.gl/qNmjZ

Answers

Exercise 12-1: *Select all that apply*

The functions of the parish nurse include:

☐ Financial advisor

☐ Guardian

☒ **Personal health counseling**

☒ **Health education**

☐ Direct patient care

☒ **Liaison with social service agencies**

☐ Legal advisor

☒ **Facilitator**

☒ **Pastoral care**

☒ **Advocate**

Exercise 12-2: *Multiple-choice question*

The best response for Johanna to give is

A. "It's only been a week; why not keep the boys a little longer until the parents come back."—NO, this is neglectful.

B. "You should go to the police and file a missing persons report for Martin and Madeline."—NO, they are not actually missing.

C. **"This is neglect, a form of child abuse, and by law must be reported to the authorities."—YES**

D. "Do you have the phone numbers of any of the Williams' friends and relatives? Let's try calling them."—NO, this is wasting valuable time.

Exercise 12-3: *True or false*

Since Alice is a responsible adult and is caring for Mark and Steve, Johanna has an ethical but not legal responsibility to report the situation.

A. True

B. **False, legally it must be reported.**

Exercise 12-4: *Fill-in*

If Johanna suspects child abuse, what else should she be assessing? What other signs and symptoms would indicate abuse?

Johanna can see evidence of neglect—boys are underweight, clothes are old and worn and too small. In addition, they were abandoned by their primary caregivers (parents). Other signs and symptoms of child abuse to assess for include physical abuse, emotional abuse, and sexual abuse.

Exercise 12-5: *Fill-in*

List the behavior changes to watch for in children that can provide clues about abuse.

Table 12-2

Behavior Changes Associated With Abuse	
Physical abuse	• Unexplained burns, bites, bruises, broken bones, or black eyes • Fading bruises or other marks noticeable after an absence from school • Seems frightened of the parents and protests or cries when it is time to go home • Shrinks at the approach of adults • Reports injury by a parent or another adult caregiver
Neglect	• Is frequently absent from school • Begs or steals food or money • Lacks needed medical or dental care, immunizations, or glasses • Is consistently dirty and has severe body odor • Lacks sufficient clothing for the weather • Abuses alcohol or other drugs • States that there is no one at home to provide care
Sexual abuse	• Has difficulty walking or sitting • Suddenly refuses to change for gym or to participate in physical activities • Reports nightmares or bedwetting • Experiences a sudden change in appetite • Demonstrates bizarre, sophisticated, or unusual sexual knowledge or behavior • Becomes pregnant or contracts a venereal disease, particularly if under age 14 • Runs away • Reports sexual abuse by a parent or another adult caregiver

Table 12-2 (*Continued*)

Behavior Changes Associated With Abuse	
Emotional abuse	• **Shows extremes in behavior, such as overly compliant or demanding behavior, extreme passivity, or aggression** • **Is either inappropriately adult (parenting other children, for example) or inappropriately infantile (frequently rocking or head-banging, for example)** • **Is delayed in physical or emotional development** • **Has attempted suicide** • **Reports a lack of attachment to the parent**

Exhibit 12-1: Answer Details

Child Welfare Information Gateway, 2007. Available from http://www.childwelfare.gov/pubs/factsheets/signs.cfm

Exercise 12-6: *Select all that apply*

Which of the following would be utilized as primary prevention strategies for child abuse or neglect?

☒ **Teenage pregnancy prevention programs**

☒ **Parenting classes**

❏ Reporting requirements

☒ **Family strengthening programs**

☒ **Community awareness**

❏ Incarceration

Exercise 12-7: *Fill-in*

What would be the most important element to assess in the home environment?

The most important element to assess in the home environment is safety.

Exercise 12-8: *Fill-in*

What strategies would the nurse consider to develop a trusting relationship during the first home visit?

Key strategies include:

• **Treat client with respect**

• **Be flexible**

• **Keep promises**

• **Listen actively**

• **Pay attention to nonverbal communication; body language—both yours and the client's**

- Be "present" and actively engaged—focus on the client
- Deal with the issue that is uppermost on the client's mind—not what is on your agenda

Exercise 12-9: *Fill-in*

What should be included in a client contract?

Client contract should include setting a short-term goal and a long-term goal; plan for every visit to progress toward goals; explain that home health services are time limited; goal is to be independent and responsible for own care (either client independently or with caregiver support); actions that facilitate and encourage self-care behaviors. Client and caregiver teaching is a priority.

Exercise 12-10: *Multiple-choice question*

The best response to Nadia's question is:

A. "It doesn't matter when he takes his medication, just as long as he takes the same time each day."—NO, this is not true.
B. "It is best that he takes his medication after he has eaten something."—YES, but this is not the only correct answer
C. "You should check his heart rate every morning before he takes this medication."—YES
D. B and C—YES.
E. All of the above—NO, not A.

Exercise 12-11: *Fill-in*

When assessing a patient following a head injury, what should Ferne consider?

- **Vital signs**
- **Level of consciousness**
- **Pupillary response**
- **Motor function or numbness**
- **Memory of events surrounding the injury**
- **Extent of injuries sustained in the fall**

Exercise 12-12: *Fill-in*

What environmental factors or modifications should be considered to reduce the risk of falling?

- **ensure adequate lighting**
- **remove throw rugs**
- **keep pathways clear of clutter**
- **ensure proper footwear that supports and contributes to balance; soles are nonslip materials**
- **proper use of assistive devices such as walkers and canes**
- **place frequently needed items within reach**

Exercise 12-13: *Select all that apply*

Which of the following statements about elder abuse are correct?

☒ **Elder abuse can be physical, verbal, financial, or psychological/emotional.**

❏ Elder abuse is a major public health problem, occurring in approximately 30% to 40% of the elderly population.

❏ The majority of elder abuse is committed by nonfamilial caregivers.

☒ **Elder abuse is underreported.**

Exercise 12-14: *Fill-in*

What should be included in a nursing assessment for elder abuse?

* **Bruises on upper arms (indicating being grabbed)**
* **Broken bones (caused from falls after being pushed)**
* **Dehydration or malnourishment**
* **Overmedication**
* **Poor physical hygiene, improper or insufficient medical care**
* **Change in behavior**
* **Withdrawn behavior, expressing feelings of helplessness or hopelessness**
* **Demanding, belligerent, or aggressive behavior**
* **Repeated trips to clinic or health care facility for injuries and falls**
* **Evidence of misuse of finances by caregivers**

Exercise 12-15: *Fill-in*

What strategies would the nurse consider to develop a trusting and supportive relationship with Nadia?

Key strategies include:

* **Pay attention to nonverbal communication; body language—both yours and Nadia's**
* **Be nonjudgmental**
* **Treat Nadia with respect**
* **Listen actively**
* **Be "present" and actively engaged—focus on Nadia**

Exercise 12-16: *Multiple-choice question*

How should Ferne respond?

A. "What you did is elder abuse and is against the law."—NO, this is accusatory.

B. Ferne should not confront Nadia. She should leave and report the incident to the authorities—NO, this is leaving the client in danger.

C. **"Caregiving is hard. There is help available that can lighten the load for you."—YES, this offers a solution.**

D. "You should reach out to your church to get some help in caring for Victor."—NO, this is passing the buck.

Exercise 12-17: *Fill-in*

What are the nursing care priorities and interventions?

- **ensure that Victor is safe in his current living situation**
- **establish trust and rapport with Victor and Nadia**
- **document factual, objective statements about Victor's condition, injuries, and interactions**
- **monitor and report suspected abuse to the appropriate local or state authorities**
- **arrange for community resources to provide additional support, assistance with activities of daily living, respite care, adult day care, and so forth**
- **continue with nursing visits**
- **refer Nadia to counseling for stress management**
- **connect Nadia with caregiver support group**

Exercise 12-18: *Multiple-choice question*

Doing blood pressure screenings at the health fair is:

A. Primary prevention—NO, this is decreasing risk factors that are modifiable.

B. **Secondary prevention—YES**

C. Tertiary prevention—NO, this is treating.

D. Health promotion—NO.

Exercise 12-19: *Fill-in*

What factors should be considered when selecting patient education material?

- **Reading level**
- **Visual appeal**
- **Information presented clearly so that it is easy to understand**
- **No jargon**
- **Culturally appropriate**

Exercise 12-20: *Select all that apply*

The World Health Organization has published guidelines regarding screening tests and strongly urges that screenings are conducted only when there is demonstrated value in doing so. These criteria include which of the following:

☒ **Screenings should be done only for diseases with serious consequences so that there is a clear health benefit.**

☒ **There must be a sufficiently reliable and safe test method.**

❑ Screenings must occur on a regular basis in order to prevent disease (screenings do not *prevent* disease, screenings permit *early detection* and *early treatment*).

☒ **There must be an effective treatment proven to be more successful when started before symptoms occur.**

☒ **There should be neutral information available so that individuals can decide for themselves whether or not to have a screening test.**

Exercise 12-21: *Fill-in*

What should Monica do next?

Monica should ask Veronica the following questions:

- **I notice you have a number of bruises; did someone do this to you?**
- **Are you afraid at home? Do you have a safety plan?**

She should offer her information regarding domestic abuse, particularly hotline information.

Exercise 12-22: *Select all that apply*

Monica knows that frequently a woman will remain in an abusive relationship because she believes that

☒ **her partner will change**

☒ **she is partly to blame for the abuse**

☒ **if she leaves, he will escalate the abuse**

☒ **she has no place to go**

☒ **she can help her abuser**

Exercise 12-23: *Fill-in*

What can Monica say to communicate caring and support for Veronica?

- **Pay attention to nonverbal communication; body language. Be nonjudgmental.**
- **Treat Veronica with respect; convey to her that she deserves to be treated with respect.**
- **Listen actively.**
- **Reassure Veronica that she is not to blame for being battered or mistreated and she is not the cause of his behavior.**
- **Convey concern about her safety.**

Exercise 12-24: *Fill-in*

What should be included in a safety plan?

- **a packed bag (ready to go)**
- **extra set of car and house keys (hidden outside in case you need to leave in a hurry)**
- **important papers**
- **have a planned safe place to go**
- **important phone numbers**

References

American Association of Colleges of Nursing. (2008). *Tool kit of resources for cultural competent education for baccalaureate nurses.* Author. Retrieved from http://www.aacn.nche.edu/education-resources/toolkit.pdf

American Nurses Association. (2004). *Nursing: Scope and standards of practice.* Silver Spring, MD: Author.

American Nurses Association. (2007). *Public health nursing: Scope and standards of practice.* Silver Spring, MD: Author.

American Nurses Association. (2010). *Nursing: Scope and standards of practice* (2nd ed.). Silver Spring, MD: Nursebooks.org

Anderson, M. (2008). *Surveillance systems focus on field epidemiology, 5*(6). North Carolina Center for Public Health Preparedness: The North Carolina Institute for Public Health. Retrieved from http://cphp.sph.unc.edu/focus/vol5/issue6/5-6SurveillanceSystems_issue.pdf

Atherton, J. S. (2011). *Learning and teaching; Knowles' andragogy: An angle on adult learning* [Online: UK]. Retrieved from http://www.learningandteaching.info/learning/knowlesa.htm

Bethell, C., Simpson, L., Stumbo, S., Carle, A. C., & Gombojav, N. (2010). National, state, and local disparities in childhood obesity. *Health Affairs, 29*(3), 347–356.

Campbell, C. (2001) *Health education behavior models and theories: A review of the literature-part I.* Mississippi State University Extension Services. Retrieved from http://msucares.com/health/health/appa1.htm

Campinha-Bacote, J. (2008). The Process of Cultural Competence in the Delivery of Healthcare Services: A Model of Care. Transcultural C.A.R.E. Associates, Available: http://www.transculturalcare.net

Centers for Disease Control and Prevention. (2003). *Report to congress on mild traumatic brain injury in the United States: Steps to prevent a serious public health problem.* Atlanta, GA: Centers for Disease Control and Prevention, National Center for Injury Prevention and Control.

Centers for Disease Control and Prevention Division of Adolescent and School Health. (2005a). *School health index: A self-assessment and planning guide.* Author. Retrieved from http://www.cdc.gov/healthyyouth/SHI/pdf/Elementary.pdf

Centers for Disease Control and Prevention. (2005b). Controlling tuberculosis in the United States: Recommendations from the American Thoracic Society, CDC, and the Infectious Diseases Society of America. *MMWR Recommendations and Reports, 54*(RR12), 1–81. Retrieved from http://www.cdc.gov/mmwr/preview/mmwrhtml/rr5412a1.htm

Centers for Disease Control and Prevention. (2007). *Excite resource library: Glossary of epidemiology terms.* Retrieved from http://www.cdc.gov/excite/library/glossary.htm

Centers for Disease Control and Prevention. (2009). *The social-ecological model: A framework for prevention* [Online]. Retrieved from http://www.cdc.gov/ViolencePrevention/overview/social-ecologicalmodel.html

Centers for Disease Control and Prevention. (2011a). *Seasonal influenza: Questions and answers.* Centers for Disease Control and Prevention, National Center for Immunization and Respiratory Diseases (NCIRD). Retrieved from http://www.cdc.gov/flu/about/qa/disease.htm

Centers for Disease Control and Prevention Division of Tuberculosis Elimination. (2011b). *Staying on track with TB medicine.* Author. Retrieved from http://www.cdc.gov/tb/publications/pamphlets/TB_trtmnt.pdf

Centers for Disease Control and Prevention Division of Tuberculosis Elimination. (2011c). *Tuberculosis (TB) fact sheets.* Author. Retrieved from http://www.cdc.gov/tb/publications/factsheets/testing/diagnosis.htm

Centers for Disease Control and Prevention. (2011d). Mental illness surveillance among adults in the United States. *Morbidity and Mortality Weekly Report (MMWR), 60*(03), 1–32 [Online]. Retrieved from http://www.cdc.gov/mmwr/preview/mmwrhtml/su6003a1.htm?s_cid=su6003a1_w

Centers for Disease Control and Prevention Division of Tuberculosis Elimination. (2012a). *Tuberculosis (TB) fact sheets.* Author. Retrieved from http://www.cdc.gov/tb/publications/factsheets/treatment/LTBItreatmentoptions.htm

Centers for Disease Control and Prevention Division of Tuberculosis Elimination. (2012b). *Tuberculosis (TB) fact sheets.* Author. Retrieved from http://www.cdc.gov/tb/publications/factsheets/treatment/treatmentHIVnegative.htm

Child Welfare Information Gateway. (2007). *Recognizing child abuse and neglect: Signs and symptoms* [Online]. Administration for Children and Families, U.S. Department of Health and Human Services. Retrieved from http://www.childwelfare.gov/pubs/factsheets/signs.cfm

Chung, J. (2006, August 29). Hispanic paradox: Income may be lower but health better than most. *The Seattle Times* [Online]. Retrieved from http://seattletimes.com/html/nationworld/2003233307_hispanichealth29.html

Community. (2012). In *Merriam-Webster.com.* Retrieved from http://www.merriam-webster.com/dictionary/community

Community. (2013). *The American Heritage® dictionary of the English language* (4th ed.).Retrieved from Dictionary.com website: http://dictionary.reference.com/browse/influence

Community. (2013). *Oxford dictionaries.* Oxford University Press. Retrieved from http://oxforddictionaries.com/definition/english/community

Council on School Health. (2008). Role of the school nurse in providing school health services. *Pediatrics, 121,* 1052. doi:10.1542/peds.2008-0382

DeWalt, D. A., Callahan, L. F., Hawk, V. H., Broucksou, K. A., Hink, A., Rudd, R., & Brach, C. (2010). *Health literacy universal precautions toolkit* (Prepared by North Carolina Network Consortium, The Cecil G. Sheps Center for Health Services Research, The University of North Carolina at Chapel Hill, under Contract No. HHSA290200710014. AHRQ Publication No. 10-0046-EF) [Online]. Rockville, MD: Agency for Healthcare Research and Quality. http://nchealthliteracy.org/toolkit/Toolkit_w_appendix.pdf

Disease Control Priorities Project. (2008). *Public health surveillance: The best weapon to avert epidemics.* Author. Retrieved from http://www.dcp2.org/file/153/dcpp-surveillance.pdf

Drabek, T. (1996, September). *The social dimensions of disaster* (FEMA Emergency Management Higher Education Project College Course Instructor Guide) [Online]. Emmitsburg, MD: Emergency Management Institute. Retrieved from http://training.fema.gov/EMIWeb/edu/completeCourses.htm

Faul, M., Xu, L., Wald, M. M., & Coronado, V. G. (2010). *Traumatic brain injury in the United States: Emergency department visits, hospitalizations, and deaths.* Atlanta, GA: Centers for Disease Control and Prevention, National Center for Injury Prevention and Control.

Gazaway, C. (2012, October 29). Train derailment, Level 3 HazMat Alert force evacuations [Online]. *Wave News.* Retrieved from http://www.wave3.com/story/19940142/ train-derailment-closes-dixie-highway-level-3-hazmat-issued

Giger, J., Davidhizar, R., Purnell, L., Harden, J., Phillips, J., & Strickland, O. (2007). American Academy of Nursing Expert panel report: Developing cultural competence to eliminate health disparities in ethnic minorities and other vulnerable populations. *Journal of Transcultural Nursing, 18*(2), 95–102.

Giger, J. N., & Davidhizar, R. E. (1991). *Transcultural Nursing: Assessment and Intervention.* St. Louis, CV Mosby. http://www.transculturalcare.net/Cultural_ Competence_Model.htm

Guttmacher Institute. (2012). *In brief fact sheet: Facts on American teens' sexual and reproductive health* [Online]. Retrieved from http://www.guttmacher.org/ pubs/FB-ATSRH.html

Hamilton, B. E., Martin, J. A., & Ventura, S. J. (2010). Births: Preliminary data for 2010. *National Vital Statistics Reports, 59*(3).

Hamilton, B. E., Martin, J. A., & Ventura, S. J. (2011). Births: Preliminary data for 2010. *National Vital Statistics Report, 60*(2), Table S-2.

HealthyPeople.gov. (2012). *About Healthy People 2020* [Online]. U.S. Department of Health and Human Services. Retrieved from http://www.healthypeople .gov/2020/about/default.aspx

Immunization Action Coalition. (2012). *Screening questionnaire for inactivated injectable influenza vaccination* (Item#P4066). Author. Retrieved from http://www .immunize.org/catg.d/p4066.pdf

Institute of Education Sciences National Center for Education Statistics. (2003). *National assessment of adult literacy (NAAL)* [Online]. http://nces.ed.gov/naal/ reading.asp

Kost, K., & Henshaw, S. (2012). *U.S. teenage pregnancies, births and abortions, 2008: National trends by age, race and ethnicity* [Online]. Guttmacher Institute. Retrieved from http://www.guttmacher.org/pubs/USTPtrends08.pdf

Lavizzo-Mourey, R. (1996). Cultural competence: Essential measurements of quality for managed care organizations. *Annals of Internal Medicine, 124*(10), 919–921.

Lewin, K. (1951). *Field theory in social science.* New York, NY: Harper & Row.

Maurer, F. A., & Smith, C. M. (2009). *Community/public health nursing practice: Health for families and populations* (4th ed.). Baltimore, MD: W. B. Saunders.

Mayer, G., & Villaire, M. (2009). Enhancing written communications to address health literacy. *The Online Journal of Issues in Nursing, 14*, doi:10.3912/OJIN .Vol14No03Man03

Mayo Clinic. (2011). *Post-traumatic stress disorder (PTSD)* [Online]. Author. Retrieved from http://www.mayoclinic.com/health/post-traumatic-stress-disorder/DS00246/ DSECTION=symptoms

Merriam-Webster Incorporated. (2012). *Merriam-Webster dictionary.* Retrieved from http://www.merriam-webster.com

Montana Public Health Department. (n.d.). *Public health nursing manual.* State of Montana.

Morbidity and Mortality Weekly Report. (2001). Recommendations for blood lead screening of young children enrolled in Medicaid: Targeting a group at high risk (Vol. 49, No. RR14, pp. 1–13). Retrieved from http://www.cdc.gov/mmwr/preview/mmwrhtml/rr4914a1.htm

Morbidity and Mortality Weekly Report. (2005). Guidelines for the investigation of contacts of persons with infectious tuberculosis: Recommendations from the National Tuberculosis Controllers Association and CDC (Vol. 54, No. RR-15). Retrieved from http://www.cdc.gov/mmwr/pdf/rr/rr5415.pdf

Morgan, N., (2010) Wound Assessment: The Basic's, Wound Care Education Institute Available: http://goo.gl/uWS9F

National Center for Environmental Health. (2011, March). *Core functions of public health and how they relate to the 10 essential environmental health services.* Retrieved from http://www.cdc.gov/nceh/ehs/ephli/core_ess.htm

National Highway Institute. (n.d.). *Principles of adult learning & instructional systems design in NIH instructor development course* [Online]. Retrieved from http://www.nhi.fhwa.dot.gov/downloads/freebies/172/PR%20Pre-course%20Reading%20Assignment.pdf

National Library of Medicine. (2012). *Wireless information system for emergency responders* [Online]. Retrieved from http://wiser.nlm.nih.gov

The National Literacy Act of 1991, Pub. L No. 102-73.

1918 flu pandemic. (2012). The History Channel website. Retrieved from http://www.history.com/topics/1918-flu-pandemic

Nilsen, M (n.d.) Hospital Guidelines, NYC DOHMH Bureau of TB Control p. 10 available: http://www.nyc.gov/html/doh/downloads/pdf/tb/tb-conf-tbhosguide.pdf

NursingPlanet.com. (2012, January 31). *Health promotion model, nursing theories: A companion to nursing theories and models* [Online]. http://nursingplanet.com/health_promotion_model.html

NYC Department of Health and Mental Hygiene, Bureau of TB Control. (n.d.). *TB manual: Section VII.* Author. Retrieved from http://www.nyc.gov/html/doh/downloads/pdf/tb/tb-manual-section7.pdf

Occupational Safety and Health Administration. (n.d.). *Noise and hearing conservation.* Retrieved from http://www.osha.gov/dts/osta/otm/noise/health_effects/index.html#effects

Pender, N. J. (1996). *Health Promotion Model.* Retrieved from http://hdl.handle.net/2027.42/85351

Queensland Occupational Therapy Fieldwork Collaborative. (2007). Adult learning theory and principles. In *The clinical educator's resource kit* [Online]. Retrieved from http://www.qotfc.edu.au/resource/index.html

Redding, C. A., Rossi, J. S., Rossi, S. R., Velicer, W. F., & Prochaska, J. O. (2000). Health behavior models [Special Issue]. *The International Electronic Journal of Health Education, 3,* 180–193. Retrieved from http://www.iejhe.siu.edu

Singh, S., & Darroch, J. E. (2000). Adolescent pregnancy and childbearing: Levels and trends in developed countries. *Family Planning Perspectives, 32*(1), 14–23.

The American Red Cross. (2013). *What we do.* Author. Available: http://www.redcross.org/what-we-do

United Nations. (2008). *Demographic yearbook*. Table 10. Retrieved from http://unstats. un.org/unsd/demographic/products/dyb2008.htm

U.S. Department of Health and Human Services. (1895). *In consensus conference on the essentials of public health nursing practice and education: Report of the conference 1985*. Rockville, MD: Author.

U.S. Department of Health and Human Services. (2008, October 28). *The Secretary's Advisory Committee on National Health Promotion and Disease Prevention Objectives for 2020. Phase I report: Recommendations for the framework and format of Healthy People 2020. Section IV. Advisory Committee findings and recommendations*. Retrieved from http://healthypeople.gov/2020/about/ advisory/PhaseI.pdf

U.S. Department of Health and Human Services, Healthy People 2020. (2012). *Nutrition and weight status*. Retrieved from http://www.healthypeople.gov/2020/topics objectives2020/overview.aspx?topicid=29#eight

U.S. Department of Health and Human Services Office of Disease Prevention and Health Promotion. (2012, October 28). *Quick guide to health literacy* [Online]. Retrieved from http://www.health.gov/communication/literacy/quickguide/ default.htm

University of Vermont. (1997, December 9). *How to collect information about your community . . . or anyone's community*. Retrieved from http://www.uvm.edu/ crs/?Page=resources/data_collection.html&SM=resources/resourcessubmenu. html

Wellington-Dufferin-Guelph Public Health. (2012, April 18). *Let's start a conversation about health and not talk about health care at all* [Video file]. Retrieved from http://youtu.be/jbqKcOqoyoo

World Health Organization. (1946). Preamble to the Constitution of the World Health Organization as adopted by the International Health Conference, New York, June 19–22, 1946; signed on July 22, 1946 by the representatives of 61 States (Official Records of the World Health Organization, No. 2, p. 100), and entered into force on April 7, 1948.

World Health Organization. (1984). *Health promotion: A discussion document*. Copenhagen: Author.

World Health Organization. (2011, September). *Non-communicable diseases fact sheet*. Retrieved from http://www.who.int/mediacentre/factsheets/fs355/en/index.html

World Health Organization. (2012a). *Health impact assessment (HIA), determinants of health*. Author. Retrieved from http://www.who.int/hia/evidence/doh/en

World Health Organization. (2012b). *Public health surveillance*. Retrieved from http:// www.who.int/topics/public_health_surveillance/en

Index